D1403413

A Parent's Guide to
CLEFT LIP
AND PALATE

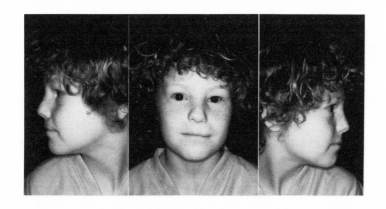

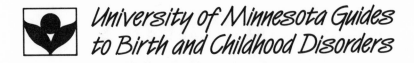

University of Minnesota Guides to Birth and Childhood Disorders

Edited by Robert J. Gorlin
Regents Professor of Oral Pathology and Genetics,
and Professor of Pediatrics, University of Minnesota

Advisory Board

David M. Brown, dean, Medical School, University of Minnesota

Judith G. Hall, Medical Genetics, University of British Columbia

Luanna H. Meyer, Special Education and Rehabilitation, Syracuse University

Margaret O'Dougherty, Neurology, Children's Hospital, Columbus, Ohio

Paul Quie, Pediatrics, University of Minnesota

Maynard Reynolds, Special Education Program, Educational Psychology, University of Minnesota

Muriel B. Ryden, School of Nursing, University of Minnesota

Joe Leigh Simpson, Clinical Genetics, Obstetrics and Gynecology, University of Tennessee, Memphis

Joseph Warshaw, Pediatrics, Yale Medical School, New Haven

Subjects of Forthcoming Volumes

Cerebral palsy	Leukemia	Spine deformities
Cystic fibrosis	Sickle-cell anemia	
Kidney disorders	and thalassemia	

A Parent's Guide to
CLEFT LIP
AND PALATE

Karlind T. Moller, Ph.D., professor and director, Cleft Palate Maxillofacial Clinic and Craniofacial Anomalies Clinic, Division of Pediatric Dentistry, Department of Preventive Sciences, School of Dentistry, University of Minnesota

Clark D. Starr, Ph.D., professor, Department of Communication Disorders, and speech pathologist, Cleft Palate Maxillofacial Clinic, University of Minnesota

and

Sylvia A. Johnson, science writer

University of Minnesota Press, Minneapolis

REMOVED FROM COLLECTION

WEST ISLIP PUBLIC LIBRARY
3 HIGBIE LANE
WEST ISLIP, NEW YORK 11795

Copyright © 1990 by the Regents of the University of Minnesota
All rights reserved. No part of this publication may be reproduced,
stored in a retrieval system, or transmitted, in any form or by any
means, electronic, mechanical, photocopying, recording, or otherwise,
without the prior written permission of the publisher.

Published by the University of Minnesota Press
2037 University Avenue Southeast, Minneapolis MN 55414
Printed in the United States of America.

Library of Congress Cataloging-in-Publication Data

Moller, Karlind T.
    A parent's guide to cleft lip and palate / Karlind T. Moller,
Clark D. Starr, and Sylvia A. Johnson.
        p.   cm. — (University of Minnesota guides to birth and
childhood disorders)
        Bibliography: p.
        Includes index.
        ISBN 0-8166-1491-1
        1. Cleft lip—Popular works.   2. Cleft palate—Popular works.
I. Starr, Clark D.   II. Johnson, Sylvia A.   III. Title.   IV. Series.
RD524.M65   1989
618.92'097522—dc20   89-5114
                                                                     CIP

The University of Minnesota
is an equal-opportunity
educator and employer.

CONTENTS

Foreword *Robert Gorlin*   vii

Preface   xi

Chapter 1.   **What Is Cleft Lip and Palate?**   5

Chapter 2.   **A Team Approach to a Complex Problem**   13

Chapter 3.   **Closing the Gap: Surgical Repair of Clefts**   19

Chapter 4.   **Feeding a Child with a Cleft**   39

Chapter 5.   **Ear Problems: Why They Happen and
             What Can Be Done about Them**   45

Chapter 6.   **Clefts and the Development of Teeth**   55

Chapter 7.   **Staying in Touch: How Clefts Affect Speech**   75

Chapter 8. The Image in the Mirror: How Clefts Affect
            Social and Psychological Development   99

Chapter 9. Can This Happen Again? The Importance
            of Genetic Counseling   105

Chapter 10. A Final Word—Optimism   111

            Glossary   115

            Helpful Organizations   119

            Suggested Reading   123

            Index   125

FOREWORD

A Parent's Guide to Cleft Palate is a volume in a series addressing the needs not only of parents but also of physicians and persons concerned with the care of children with relatively common disorders. We used as a model *The Child with Down's Syndrome*, written by David W. Smith, M.D., and Ann Asper Wilson and first published in 1973 by W. B. Saunders, Philadelphia. The book is very valuable because it makes the complex concepts of genetics and pediatrics understandable to parents. Such is the goal of our series.

In *A Parent's Guide to Cleft Palate*, it was the authors' intent to provide parents and other health-care givers with a knowledgeable discussion of the nature and causes of cleft lip and cleft palate together with information about the medical, dental, speech, hearing, and psychosocial concerns. They discuss current methods of treatment and the desirability of a team approach to a child with a cleft in carrying out treatment over the many years of care. They cover the surgical repair of clefts and the ideal times for surgery. They deal with very special problems such as how to feed a baby with a cleft, how to cope with middle-ear infections, and what can be done for unusual speech. They review the orthodontic aspects of facial clefting and genetic counseling.

This book is written by Karlind T. Moller, Ph.D., Clark D. Starr, Ph.D., and Sylvia A. Johnson. Karlind T. Moller is presently professor in Pediatric Dentistry and Communication Disorders and director of the Cleft Palate Maxillofacial and Craniofacial Clinics at the University of Minnesota, Minneapolis, Minnesota. He is indeed a Minnesota product, having received his B.S., M.A., and Ph.D. in Communication Disorders from the University of Minnesota. Dr. Moller received the award for Outstanding Clinical Achievement for the American Speech and Hearing Association. He has been active in the American Speech, Language and Hearing Association and the American Cleft Palate Association. Clark D. Starr is professor of Communication Disorders at the University of Minnesota. He earned his Ph.D. at Northwestern University at Evanston, Illinois and also served as director of the Speech and Hearing Clinic at the University of Minnesota. Additionally, he was chair of the Department of Communication Disorders at the University of Minnesota. Dr. Starr is past president of the Minnesota Speech, Language and Hearing Association. I have had the good fortune to know both Dr. Moller and Dr. Starr for over twenty years as respected colleagues. Their sensitivity to parents' problems is legendary. Sylvia A. Johnson is an award-winning editor and writer of books for young people. She received an M.A. in English from the University of Illinois. Ms. Johnson has collaborated with writers in the fields of anthropology, archaeology, botany, behavioral biology, entomology, and psychiatry.

The need for this series is obvious. Parents of a child with a serious disability need answers. They need to know not only the nature of their child's disorder but also its possible causes, its prognosis, the limitations it will impose on the child, the impact it will have on the entire family, and the chances of it recurring in either the parents' future children or in the affected child's children. It is also important that parents be informed about community resources that can help them deal with the disorder. And, certainly, they need to know what they themselves can do to help.

In spite of good intentions, the health professional has not always been an effective communicator. These books are designed to open the lines of communication between the health professional and parents by increasing parents' understanding and providing them with a basic vocabulary for easier and more accurate expression of the worries, doubts, and uncertainties attendant to each disorder. It is our intention that health professionals play a vital part by supplementing each text with their own expertise. We cannot hope to answer all the questions that may be posed by parents, but we believe that each book will go a long way in answering many of the common ones.

R. J. G.

PREFACE

As the parent of a child with a cleft lip or palate you may believe that you and your family are victims of a serious misfortune. This birth defect is an obvious one that can be seen, felt, and heard. When you first learned that your child had a cleft, you probably felt many conflicting emotions: anger, shock, disbelief, disappointment, sadness, guilt, confusion, fear. Perhaps you were overwhelmed by what had happened to you. How could something that was expected to make you feel so good produce so many bad feelings? That perfect child that you had planned on was not perfectly normal.

No doubt you were also very concerned about your baby's future. What would he or she look like? How would the cleft affect the growth of teeth and the development of speech? Would you as a parent be able to provide the care needed by a child with such a defect?

All these feelings and concerns are very natural. They are shared by most parents of children born with disorders, including cleft lip and palate. In facing your situation, it is important not to deny any negative feelings you may have. Admitting such feelings to yourself and discussing them with family members and with professionals are necessary to the process of understanding and adjustment.

Although it is important not to deny negative feelings like guilt, fear, and anger, it is also important not to be overwhelmed by them. We firmly believe that many of the negative feelings that parents have about clefts result from lack of information or wrong information. The purpose of this book is to provide the information that will help you to better understand your child's condition: its nature, cause, and treatment. The more that you learn about your child's cleft, the more you will realize that there is every reason for optimism.

Parents of children born with cleft lip or palate may think their situation is very special, but they are certainly not alone. In fact, clefts are among the most common birth defects. In the United States, approximately 5,000 children are born each year with this kind of malformation—about one child in every 600 to 700 births. The rate of occurrence is about the same in Canada, Great Britain, and other countries with predominantly white populations. Statistics show that clefts are most common among Native Americans, somewhat more common among Japanese and Chinese children, and somewhat less common among blacks.

Another important fact you should know about cleft lip and palate is that it is a birth defect that responds very well to treatment. There are many well-established techniques for repairing the opening in your child's lip or palate and for dealing with the other problems caused by the condition. This treatment is complex and cannot be done overnight. The important thing to remember is that it can be very successful in correcting the defect. Given the appropriate care, your child has every chance of living a normal life.

This book provides basic information about the medical condition of cleft lip and palate, and the common methods used to treat it. It will help you to better understand the problem and to gain the knowledge that will enable you to become actively involved in your child's treatment.

A Parent's
Guide to
CLEFT LIP
AND PALATE

Chapter 1
WHAT IS CLEFT
LIP AND PALATE?

The word *cleft* commonly refers to a "split" or "separation," and that is exactly what a cleft lip or palate is. People with this medical condition have a split in the upper lip (sometimes extending into the floor of the nose), in the upper bony gum ridge, or in the roof of the mouth (palate). In some cases, the split occurs in all these areas. What has happened is that sections of skin, muscle, and bone normally joined have been separated by a cleft. It is important to understand that nothing is missing in a person with a cleft; all the parts of the normal mouth are there, but they are divided instead of being fused.

These separations are, in fact, part of the normal prenatal development of all humans. Each child growing inside its mother's body goes through a stage during which clefts exist in the developing lip and palate. At about the fourth week after conception takes place, the human embryo has splits or clefts in the region usually referred to as the *primary palate*, made up of the upper lip and gum ridge. The clefts are on both sides of the upper lip and extend into the area that will eventually develop into the nostrils (Figure 1). By the seventh week, the two sides of the lip as well as the gum ridge normally come together and merge, forming a partition between the front parts of the nose and the mouth.

During this same early period of development, clefts also exist in the roof of the mouth (Figure 2). This area, known as

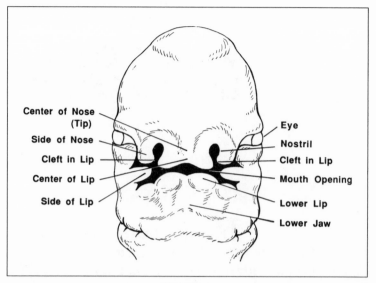

FIGURE 1

Head of developing embryo at approximately four weeks. Early in an embryo's development, clefts exist on both sides of the upper lip and extend up into the area of the nose.

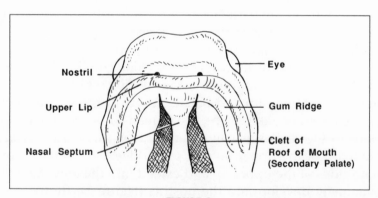

FIGURE 2

Roof of mouth of developing embryo at approximately seven weeks (view from below). By the seventh week, the clefts in the lip and gum ridge (the primary palate) have closed, but clefts still exist in the roof of the mouth (the secondary palate). The bony partition in the nose, known as the nasal septum, can be seen between the two clefts.

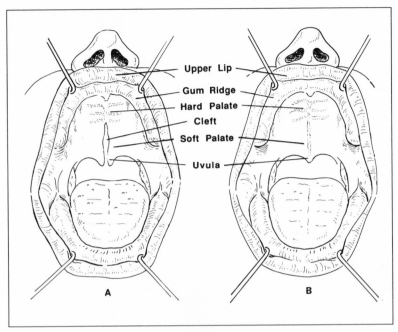

FIGURE 3

Closing of the secondary palate at approximately ten weeks (A) and twelve weeks (B). (A) shows the partial closing of the hard palate that has taken place by approximately the tenth week of prenatal development. By the twelfth week, the hard and soft palate and the uvula are completely closed, as shown in (B).

the *secondary palate,* includes the hard and soft parts of the roof of the mouth (the hard and soft palates) and the uvula (that little piece of tissue hanging down at the back of the mouth). By approximately the tenth to the twelfth week, the clefts in the secondary palate close, completing the normal separation between the nose and mouth from the front all the way back to the tip of the uvula. Figure 3 pictures two stages in the closing of the secondary palate, and Figure 4 shows the results of normal lip and nose merging. Figure 5 is a view from below showing all the normal mouth structures.

In a child born with cleft lip or palate, something has obviously happened to interfere with the normal development of the primary and secondary palates. For reasons not yet

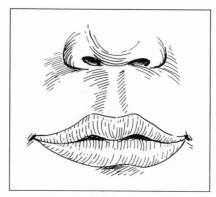

FIGURE 4
The lip and nose when normal merging has taken place.

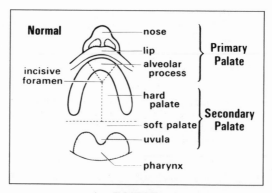

FIGURE 5
The normal nose, lip, and mouth structures seen from below. This drawing shows the primary and secondary palates, two general regions of the mouth often referred to in describing clefts. The primary palate includes the lip and gum ridge back to a spot called the incisive foramen. Behind this spot is the secondary palate, made up of the hard and soft palates and the uvula. The dashed lines indicate the areas where clefts occur.

clearly understood, the fusion of some or all of the mouth parts did not occur. The resulting cleft may affect only the primary palate, that is, the lip and gum ridge (Figure 6). Other clefts involve only the secondary palate (Figure 7). In 40 to 50 percent of persons with clefts, both the primary and

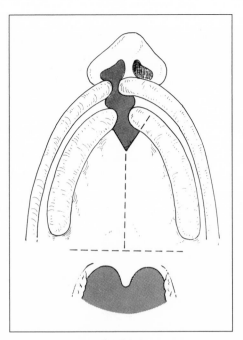

FIGURE 6
A one-sided cleft involving the primary palate only.

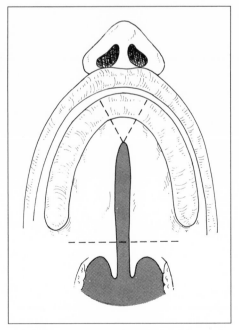

FIGURE 7
A cleft involving the secondary palate only.

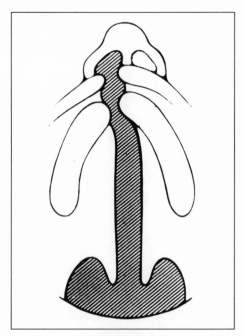

FIGURE 8
A one-sided cleft involving both the primary and secondary palates.

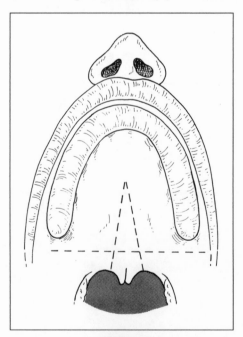

FIGURE 9
A submucous cleft. A submucous cleft affects the muscles that normally attach in the middle of the soft palate but does not affect the skin covering the roof of the mouth. Its presence is often indicated only by a small cleft in the uvula.

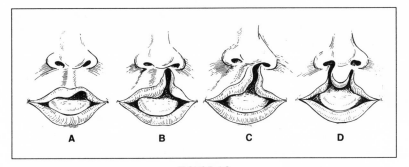

FIGURE 10
Varieties of lip clefts. (A), (B), and (C) show unilateral, or one-sided, clefts in the lip and gum ridge. A bilateral, or two-sided, cleft is seen in (D).

secondary palates are split (Figure 8). A less common kind of cleft affects the muscles in the soft palate. Known as a sub-mucuous cleft, it is often indicated only by a cleft in the uvula (Figure 9).

All of these kinds of clefts may be complete or partial, de-pending on whether they extend through all or only part of the mouth structures. Clefts affecting the lip can occur on just one side (a unilateral cleft) or on both sides (bilateral). Figure 10 shows some of the common varieties of lip clefts.

What Causes Clefting?

As you can see from the above description, we have a pretty good idea of how clefts develop. They are caused by some kind of interruption in the normal process that merges the lip, palate, and other mouth parts before birth. *Why* the merging does not take place is not so obvious. We do know that there is probably no single cause for all clefts.

In many birth defects like clefting, several factors are usu-ally involved. One of these factors is often genetic; the ab-normal development is produced by the genetic material that a child inherits from his or her parents. There may be a flaw in a single *gene* (the basic unit of heredity), or in a combination of genes, that prevents the merging of the mouth parts from taking place. Sometimes the problem is caused by defects in the *chromosomes*, which are made up of many different genes. Extra chromosomes or partially missing ones can give the wrong genetic message to the developing embryo. Other possible factors are environmental rather than genetic. Harmful agents such as drugs or infections might interfere with normal development at a critical time.

Today, most researchers think that the majority of clefts in humans are probably caused by a combination of genetic and environmental factors. A child may inherit some genetic characteristic that makes the development of a cleft possible. Unless certain environmental factors are present, however, the possibility will not become a reality. It is the chance combination of factors occurring in the same person that is probably responsible for most cases of cleft lip or palate.

This explanation for clefting is, of course, a generalization based on studies of large numbers of families with members having clefts. At the present time, the specific genetic and environmental factors involved have not been identified. Research is continuing, however, and someday answers to the puzzle may be found.

In the meantime, there is a great deal of professional help available for individuals with cleft lip and palate, and for their families. This help covers a wide range, from intricate surgery that can close clefts to genetic counseling for families concerned about having more children born with the same problem. The remaining sections of this book will describe the basic help available, the people who give it, and the results that may be expected. The vital role that parents and other caretakers play in the treatment of children with cleft lip and palate will also be discussed.

Chapter 2
A TEAM APPROACH TO A COMPLEX PROBLEM

Since clefts involve a part of the body as central to human activity as the mouth, it is not surprising that these defects can have wide-ranging effects when uncorrected. Of course, not every child with a cleft has the same set of problems. Each situation is unique, depending on the original nature of the cleft and the specific pattern of growth and development. There are, however, some general areas of concern for all children born with this defect. Following is an overview of these areas and of the ways in which the problems are usually handled. Later chapters will discuss each subject in more detail.

Clefts: The Source of All the Problems

The primary area of concern, and the source of all other potential problems, is the existence of the clefts or separations in your child's lip or palate. It should be encouraging for you to learn that these clefts can usually be repaired by surgery and that this is one of the first treatments your child will receive. The precise timing of the surgery will depend upon the child's general health, the severity of the clefts, and other factors involved in growth and development.

Generally, the lip and nose are initially repaired within

weeks after birth or at least during the first few months of the child's life. The palate is usually closed when the child is between six and eighteen months old. Following this primary surgery, further operations may be necessary to revise the shape of the lip and nose and to improve appearance and function. The surgeon who will repair your child's cleft will probably be the first medical specialist you will meet after your pediatrician or family doctor.

Difficulty in Feeding

A very early problem that may appear in caring for a child with cleft lip or palate is difficulty in feeding. Before surgical repair is completed, the split in the lip and other parts of the mouth may affect the normal action of sucking that is so vital in a child's first months of life. Research and experience have shown that there are ways to help children with clefts to drink from a bottle and later to eat solid food. Pediatricians and pediatric nurses can help new parents learn these methods so that their child can get the nourishment needed for normal growth.

Hearing Problems

You might not think that hearing would be a problem in children with clefts, but it often is. A child with a cleft palate is more susceptible than other children to inflammation of the middle ear. Such problems occurring early in life can result in some hearing loss. That is why it is important that the health of your child's ears be checked regularly by a physician, pediatrician, or ear, nose, and throat specialist (otolaryngologist). Periodic visits to an audiologist, a specialist in hearing problems, can also determine whether there is any hearing loss and, if so, its nature and extent. Ear problems in children with clefts respond very well to treatment, and they also tend to decrease with age. Nevertheless, this is an important area of concern in the early months of a child's life.

Abnormal Development of Teeth

If your child's cleft involves the alveolar process, the bony gum ridge that contains the upper teeth, you may expect some differences in the development of the teeth. All the permanent teeth may not appear, and those that do develop may not be positioned normally. The growth of your child's teeth should be carefully observed by a pediatric dentist starting at about age two. Eventually, the help of other dental specialists may be needed. An orthodontist can align or straighten the existing teeth to obtain the best possible bite and appearance. As your child grows, it may be necessary to consult an oral surgeon, a dental specialist who can surgically move the bones of the jaws and repair the cleft in the gum ridge. A prosthodontist will be able to provide bridges or partial dentures for the replacement of missing teeth.

These concerns will become important as your child's permanent teeth come in and the bones of the jaw grow to their mature size. Your primary concern during the early years will be good dental health, just as important for a child with a cleft as for other children. Care of the teeth at home and regular examinations by a dentist will make sure that your child's existing teeth and gums are strong and healthy.

Problems With Speech and Language

Like all children, a child with a cleft will begin learning about language and speech from the very first day of life. Your baby will probably also make sounds similar to those made by most babies. However, the development of normal speech habits can be affected by clefts since these defects involve the lip and palate, two parts of the mouth involved in the production of sounds. Early surgical repair of the lip and palate usually provides a much improved mechanism for speech. As your child grows, the development of speech and communication skills should be followed closely by a speech pathologist, therapist, or clinician. It is possible that the structures used to produce speech will require further surgical repair. These specialists will be able to monitor your child's progress and advise you about the need for additional surgery.

A Team Approach

All the specialists mentioned above will play a part in the care of a child with cleft lip or palate. Although the emphasis may shift from one specialist to another as your child grows and develops, all will continue to contribute throughout the years of treatment. Since surgical, dental, speech, and hearing problems are often interrelated, we strongly believe that the most effective way to ensure the best possible results is by a team approach. Such an approach involves periodic examinations, evaluations, discussion, and planning by all the team members.

In some communities, the team members who evaluate your child periodically are the same people who provide the direct care. They will discuss their findings with each other when deciding on the most appropriate treatment. In other areas, members of the interdisciplinary team are colleagues of the specialists who are treating your child in your local community. In this situation, the team's observations and recommendations will be communicated to you and to those responsible for direct care so that final decisions about treatment can be made.

In both these situations, the benefits of periodic interdisciplinary evaluation are available to the professionals involved, to you, and, most important, to your child. The result will be comprehensive diagnosis and treatment that will provide the best care available.

Chapter 3
CLOSING THE GAP: SURGICAL REPAIR OF CLEFTS

Surgery is one of the first medical treatments given to a child with cleft lip or palate. In this chapter, we will describe the nature of the surgery, its timing, and how it will affect your child's speech, appearance, and physical well-being. First, however, we would like to introduce you to the surgeon.

In most instances, your child's surgery will be done by a specialist who is a plastic surgeon, a pediatric surgeon, or an otolaryngologist. These are all medical doctors who have spent an additional three to five years in training to become surgeons. Part of their training involved learning a wide range of surgical procedures, while the rest was spent in areas of special interest. For example, the plastic surgeon specializes in doing surgery that replaces or reshapes parts of the body that have been damaged or lost because of disease, accidents, or conditions present at birth. The pediatric surgeon is interested in the general surgical needs of children, including the repair of missing or defective structures. The specialities of the otolarnygologist are problems of the ear, nose, and throat that can be corrected through surgery.

Regardless of their areas of interest and special training, all the surgeons who will treat your child have an overall concern for the problems of children with clefts. They continue to spend a great deal of time studying these problems and learning to deal with them. Fortunately, surgeons with this kind of training and concern can be found in most parts of the world where advanced medical treatment is available.

Lip Surgery

If your child has a cleft lip, the first surgery will repair it. The decision on the timing of the surgery will be based on a careful study of the child's health and development. When your baby appears to be in good health, is eating well, and is beginning to grow, surgery will be scheduled. This usually occurs sometime between the second and tenth week after birth. Your doctor will discuss the specific timing factors with you.

José Martinez was born with a unilateral cleft lip and palate. He was a healthy baby, and his parents took him home from the hospital four days after his birth. José was checked by his pediatrician once a week for the next four weeks. During that time, he gained weight, ate well, and remained generally healthy. At José's fourth checkup, the pediatrician told his parents that their son was ready for lip surgery. The Martinezes were pleased by the news and immediately made an appointment to see their surgeon. The operation was scheduled for the following week, and José's parents eagerly looked forward to the day when the cleft in their son's lip would be repaired.

In performing lip surgery, the surgeon can choose from a variety of procedures. The one used on your child will depend in part on the extent to which the lip is cleft and the amount of tissue present. In each case, the surgeon carefully studies the child's lip tissue, then makes some incisions that will allow the two lip segments to be brought together and sutured (sewn) so that the lip will look whole and normal. Figure 11 shows a typical lip cleft before and during surgery. The accompanying photographs are of a child with a unilat-

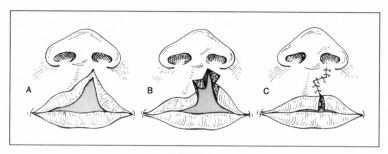

FIGURE 11
Surgical repair of a unilateral lip cleft.   To repair a unilateral lip cleft (A), the surgeon makes incisions (B) that allow the lip segments to be brought together and sutured.

eral lip cleft before and after surgery, and at age eight. It is difficult to tell that she once had a cleft.

Terry Peters was eight weeks old when he had surgery to repair the cleft in his lip. After the operation, his parents, Sid and Louise, were pleased that their son's lip was now whole, but they were concerned about the scar that the operation had left. It seemed large to them, and it was not a straight line but very irregular. Their surgeon reassured them that all surgical scars appear large at first but usually diminish with time, even though they never completely disappear. The scar from cleft lip surgery is deliberately made irregular in shape so that the tissue changes taking place after surgery, including growth of the lip tissue, will not be distorted. As the surgeon explained to the Peters, experience has shown that an irregular scar will, in the long run, produce a better appearance than a straight scar.

Terry also had a cleft in the bony alveolar ridge of his upper jaw, and this split was still there after the operation. The Peters were not surprised, since their surgeon had told them earlier that this part of the cleft would not be repaired at the same time as the lip cleft. The bony ridge in the upper jaw, from which the upper teeth develop, still had a lot of grow-

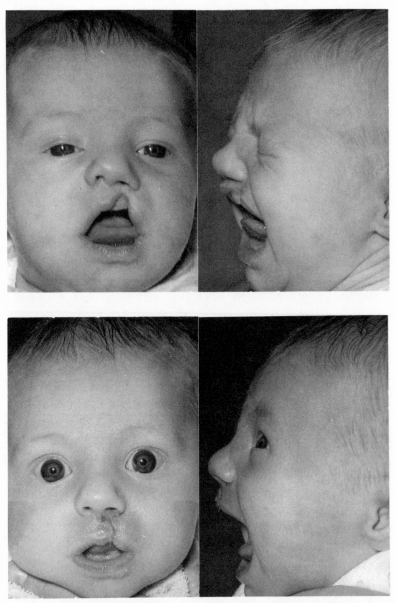

A child with a unilateral lip cleft before and after surgery.

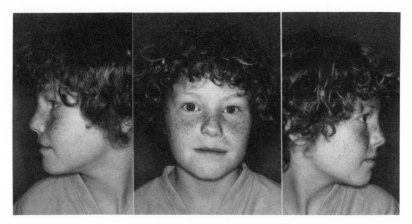

These photographs show the same child at age eight. It is hard to tell that she once had a cleft.

ing to do, and surgery might limit it from reaching its full size. The Peters knew that if it were necessary to repair the alveolar cleft, the operation would be performed later, probably sometime after Terry was five years old.

Some clefts extend through the lip up into the nose, causing the two nostrils to be different in size and shape (Figure 12). In such cases, the surgical procedure may be more complicated than that for a cleft in the lip alone. After careful study, the surgeon may find that there is not enough tissue in the two lip segments to shape an acceptable lip and nostril. The surgeon may have to create small flaps of tissue in other sections of the lip and nose, and reposition them to provide the amount of tissue needed.

This kind of surgery also leaves an irregular scar in the lip. Even after surgical repair, the nostrils may not be identical in size and shape, but with continued growth, and perhaps some additional surgery, they will become more symmetrical.

The accompanying photographs show how the child's lip cleft extended up into the nose and distorted the shape of the

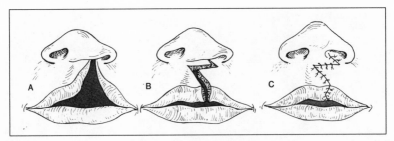

FIGURE 12
Surgical repair of a unilateral lip cleft extending into the nose. Unilateral clefts extending through the lip into the nose often cause the nostril on the cleft side to be misshapen (A). Surgery produces an appropriately shaped nostril and lip by bringing the separated segments together (B,C) or by repositioning flaps of lip and nose tissue.

nostril on the cleft side. After surgery, the lip cleft has been repaired and the nostril is more normal in appearance.

Some children have bilateral clefts, occurring on both sides of the lip and involving one nostril or both. Surgery in these cases is similar to that described above, except that the surgeon may find it necessary to close one side of the lip first and then wait several weeks before operating on the other side.

Regardless of the kind of cleft or the surgical procedure, the major effect of the initial surgery will be to make your child's face whole. After the swelling has gone down and the stitches have been removed, you will see a dramatic improvement in facial appearance, and will find it much easier to feed your child. The surgical repair of the lip clefts will also provide the improved mouth structures needed for the development of speech.

Will Additional Lip Surgery Be Necessary?

Lip surgery is done very early in a child's life. After surgery, the child will continue to grow, and with growth, the shape of the lip and the nose will change. These changes may improve your child's appearance. It is possible, however, that the changes may have the opposite effect and may create a need for additional, or secondary, surgery.

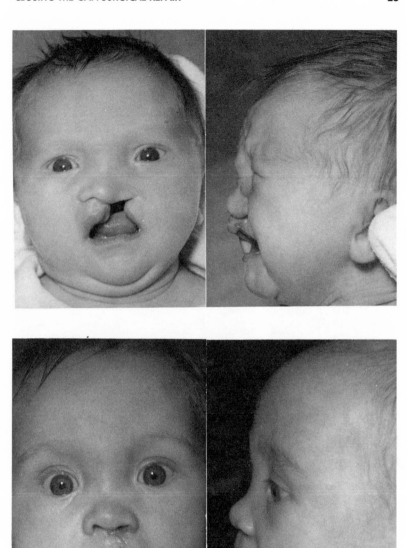

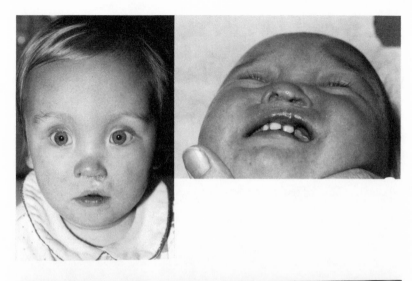

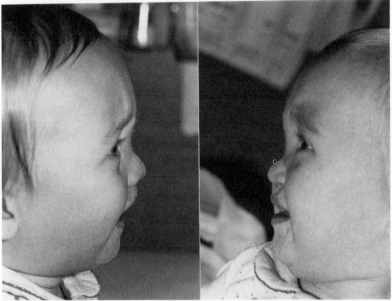

Before surgery, this child's lip cleft extended up into the nose and distorted the shape of the nostril on the cleft side. After surgery, the lip cleft has been repaired and the nostril is more normal in appearance.

One kind of problem is the uneven growth of tissue on the two sides of the lip. If this occurs, another operation may be needed to reshape the lip so that both sides are more equal. Another problem affects the line separating the reddish lip tissue from the paler tissue on the rest of the face. Sometimes initial surgery and subsequent growth result in an irregular or inappropriately shaped line between these two areas of tissue. Secondary surgery might be required to improve this situation. Growth may also increase or accentuate the difference in the size and shape of the nostrils. This, too, can often be remedied by additional surgery.

These kinds of problems influence your child's appearance, but they usually don't affect functions such as eating or speech. The scheduling of secondary surgery is usually based on a decision that your child's welfare will benefit by an improvement in appearance. For example, when a child is about to start school, parents may decide that an improved physical appearance is important to make sure that the youngster has every opportunity to participate fully in all social activities, making friends and getting along well with schoolmates. If you reach such a decision, the surgeon will study your child's physical condition—growth, development of teeth, condition of lip tissue, and other factors. Based on this evaluation, the surgeon will suggest an appropriate time for the desired surgery.

There are other occasions when secondary surgery to improve appearance may seem appropriate. A very common one is when your child becomes a teen-ager, a time of life when looks can be very important.

Cindy Corio was thirteen when she told her mother, Marie, that she was unhappy with her appearance. She had had surgery to close bilateral clefts in her lip when she was an infant. Now the shape of her lip was somewhat distorted because of uneven growth around the scars. Cindy was very self-conscious about this and felt that the other kids in school were talking about her appearance behind her back. Cindy's mother tried to tell her that she was exaggerating the strangeness of her looks and her friends' reactions, but Cindy was not convinced. When Cindy started finding excuses not to go to school—

she had a series of upset stomachs and colds—Marie Corio decided it was time to make an appointment with Cindy's surgeon to talk about the possibility of additional lip surgery.

Whenever you believe, as Marie Corio did, that your child's appearance is interfering with pyschological or social well-being, the potential for improvement through additional surgery should be investigated. As your child grows older, he or she will become more and more involved in making decisions regarding surgery. Just as you have done, your son or daughter will want to learn about the options and possible outcomes in order to make an informed decision.

There are several things you and your child might keep in mind when considering the possibility of secondary surgery. First, there are many factors that affect the way an individual gets along with others and enjoys life. Although appearance may be one of these factors, it is seldom the only one responsible for the problems we have with ourselves and others. In deciding on secondary surgery, it is important not to expect that improving physical appearance will solve all of a child's problems.

Second, surgery may improve appearance, but it does not create perfection. In discussions with your surgeon, you will be told about the limitations of the surgical procedures. You and your child should learn to have realistic expectations about the outcome of any operation.

A third thing to remember is that surgery is always a serious business. Physicans do not subject children to surgery unless they are convinced that the potential outcome warrants the risks. And there are risks in secondary lip surgery. They may be small compared to those involved in other types of surgery, but they do exist. When a child is placed under a general anesthesia and when incisions and sutures are used, there is always a possibility of problems developing. Although the risk of death is extremely low, problems can occur that affect the way surgical wounds heal and, in turn, the anticipated surgical results. Your surgeon will inform you of these risks, and you and your child should keep them in mind when deciding on secondary surgery.

Palate Surgery

The second kind of primary surgery performed on a child with cleft lip and palate is surgical closure of the hard and soft palates. This operation is usually done at about one year of age, although some surgeons prefer to wait another year or more. The surgeon must take many factors into consideration when deciding to do palatal surgery. As with lip surgery, the child must be in good health. And the child must have grown to the point where his or her mouth is large enough to allow the surgeon to work inside it. Finally, the tissue surrounding and covering the palate must have developed to the point where there is a sufficient amount to use in closing the cleft.

Once the operation has been scheduled, the surgical procedures used will depend on the type and extent of your child's cleft and your surgeon's preference for dealing with the specific problems involved. In general, the surgery will have two main goals. One will be to cover the cleft of the hard palate (the bony part of the roof of the mouth) with tissue so that no air or food can leak into the nose. The second goal will be to unite the two parts of the soft palate so that this structure can function normally. Let's take a closer look at each of these two goals.

Repairing the Cleft in the Hard Palate

If your child's cleft extends into the hard palate, the surgeon will try to close this opening by using the thin layers of tissue covering the two palatal bones. Tissue near the edge of the cleft will be partially detached from each of the palatal bones, then brought together and sutured. If the hard palate cleft is unusually wide or if there is not enough tissue on the palatal bones to allow this type of closure, the surgeon will move tissue from elsewhere in the mouth or from inside the nose and use it to cover the cleft area.

It is important to note that these procedures do not involve bringing the palatal bones together to close the cleft. Instead, they use tissue to cover the opening. Surgeons rarely operate on the bones of a young child because in doing so they might disturb future facial growth by preventing the bones from developing to their normal size. With cleft palate, there is no need to take this risk. Using softer tissue to cover the cleft is very effective in closing off the mouth from the nose and providing a thoroughly satisfactory surface for eating and speaking.

Surgery to cover the cleft in the hard palate does not involve the bone around the front edge of the palate, the alveolar ridge in which the upper teeth grow. As we have explained earlier, surgery in this area is generally not done until later, usually after the permanent teeth have begun to appear. At this early stage of life, lack of closure in the alveolar bone will not have an important effect on your child's ability to speak or eat. If there is a need for it, the alveolar cleft can be repaired later.

Repairing the Cleft in the Soft Palate

The soft palate is usually closed at the same time as the hard palate, although some surgeons prefer to do it in a separate operation. (Figure 13 shows a common procedure for making both repairs in the same operation.) Closure of the soft palate is somewhat more complex than the repair of the hard palate. The two soft palate segments must be united in a way that will allow the muscles connected to them to function properly. These muscles are called the *levators* because their job is to elevate the soft palate. They are normally attached at the midline of the palate and on each side of the throat above the palate. When the muscles contract or shorten, they lift the soft palate up to where it touches the back of the throat and its two side walls. When the palate is raised in this way, it forms a separation between the mouth and the nose.

A cleft in the soft palate prevents the levator muscles from

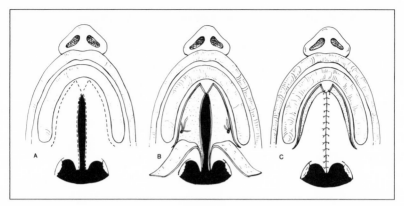

FIGURE 13
Surgical repair of the hard and soft palate. This illustration shows one of the types of surgery used to repair the hard and soft palate. Flaps of tissue from the surface of the hard palate are outlined (A) and then carefully raised (B). After the muscles of the soft palate are sutured together, the flaps are moved toward the midline of the palate and sutured (C). This procedure provides a covering for the cleft in the hard palate and joins the two parts of the soft palate.

functioning normally in raising the palate. To remedy this problem, the surgeon closes the cleft in two stages. First, the muscle ends in both segments of the palate are carefully brought together and sutured. Then the surface tissue that covers the muscles is joined.

This type of surgery, or a variation of it, usually results in a soft palate that functions properly and allows the mouth and nasal cavities to be sufficiently separated during eating and speaking. Following the operation, most children quickly learn how and when to use the palate to create this separation. Sometimes, however, a child will have difficulty learning how to use the new closure mechanism. Problems with closure most often arise in relation to speech. If your child is having this kind of problem, he or she may need some help from a speech clinician. (Chapter 7 describes these problems in more detail.)

Will Additional Palate Surgery Be Necessary?

Most often, the hard and soft palate are united success-fully in the original surgery. However, sometimes problems develop later that require secondary surgery, so it is impor-tant to know that secondary procedures are available if they are needed.

It is the soft palate that most commonly requires secondary surgery, usually because the initial repair of the cleft has not provided adequate closure between the mouth and the nose. This can happen for several different reasons. The soft palate may not be long enough to reach the back wall of the throat. Or although the palate is sufficiently long, the muscles do not elevate it enough to make contact with the back of the throat. With either of these conditions, the child may have eating problems, getting food into his or her nose and not be-ing able to suck through a straw. Inadequate closure may also cause air to leak through the nose when blowing and a nasal sound in speech. In these situations, secondary sur-gery on the soft palate may be required.

Another kind of problem with closure occurs when the palate is long enough and the muscles are able to elevate it and close off the nose from the mouth but only during cer-tain activities. For example, the palate may reach the back wall of the throat when the child swallows but not when he or she speaks. This is what happened with Danny Cohen. After the cleft in his soft palate was repaired, Danny had no problems eating, sucking, or blowing, but his speech sounded nasal. Speech therapy was recommended to solve the problem since it appeared that Danny had the physical equipment for better closure but was not able to use it appro-priately during speech. In such a situation, a speech clinician and sometimes a prosthodontist can help the child learn how to make closure for speech. Therapy was successful in cor-recting Danny's problem, so additional surgery was not needed.

Sometimes, however, therapy does not succeed, possibly because the child cannot achieve the rapid and highly con-

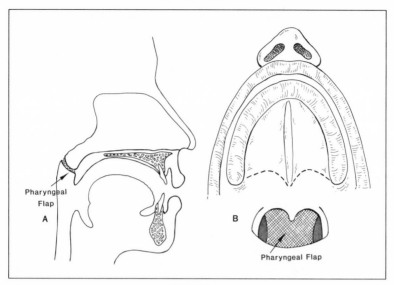

FIGURE 14

Pharyngeal flap surgery. In pharyngeal flap surgery, the surgeon creates a bridge or flap of tissue that connects the soft palate to the back wall of the throat. This flap improves closure between the nose and the mouth and helps to eliminate nasal sound in speech.

trolled closure needed for speech. In this situation, and in the others described above, secondary surgery must be performed.

The most common type of secondary surgery to improve closure on the soft palate closure is called *pharyngeal flap surgery*. This procedure is designed to take advantage of the movement of the throat (pharyngeal) walls that occurs during closure. As the soft palate is raised upward and backward to touch the throat walls, the walls themselves usually move inward to meet the rising palate.

In pharyngeal flap surgery, the surgeon makes use of this natural movement to improve closure. He or she creates a bridge of tissue, called a flap, which connects the soft palate to the back wall of the throat. Figure 14 shows how this is done. As you can see in the drawing, there is an open space on both sides of the bridge. When the child swallows, sucks, blows, or speaks, the throat walls move toward the bridge and close the openings, thus closing off the nose from the mouth. When these actions are not being performed, the spaces remain open so that the child can breathe through the nose and so that fluids from the nose can drain into the throat, as they normally do. This type of surgery works very well for most children. It is not uncomfortable and seldom causes problems.

Another type of secondary surgery is very similar to the initial surgery used to close the soft palate. In this operation, the palate is reopened, that is, the two parts are surgically divided. Before closing them, the surgeon removes a flap of tissue from the surface of the hard palate or from somewhere else in the mouth and moves it onto the soft palate. The extra tissue allows the soft palate to be lengthened so that it better reaches the back walls of the throat. This procedure, usually called *palatal lengthening* or *palatal pushback*, can be performed in several ways. When successfully completed, it makes the palate long enough to accomplish closure for eating and speaking.

Another procedure in secondary surgery involves the use of *pharyngeal augmentation* to reduce the size of the throat opening at the point where the palate touches it during closure. Instead of lengthening the palate, this approach attempts to decrease the distance that the palate has to move to accomplish closure. The implants used may be made with tissue (taken from other places in the child's body) or with artificial substances that are injected or surgically placed in the throat walls. This is only one of the techniques that have been developed recently for use in secondary palate surgery. In the future, no doubt others will be developed to help solve the problem of inadequate closure between the soft palate and the throat.

For some children initial surgery on the soft palate is successful, but there may be problems with the surgical repair of the hard palate, requiring secondary surgery. These problems usually involve a developing hole, or *fistula*, in the area where the two pieces of tissue covering the hard palate have been sutured together. Such a fistula may cause the child to get food into his or her nose while eating and to speak nasally. Although surgical repair is not a simple procedure, the hole can usually be closed with a piece of tissue taken from elsewhere in the mouth.

Nonsurgical Methods of Closing the Palate

In some situations, surgery may not be possible or successful. Some young children may not be good candidates for surgery. For example, a child may have a heart condition that cannot be treated until later in life, making palatal surgery impossible until this time. In this situation, a prosthesis can be inserted into the mouth to close it off from the nose. In other situations, a prosthesis is used as a training device when surgery has provided the potential for adequate closure, but the palatal muscles need to be developed to function properly in raising the soft palate.

Devices used to achieve closure are usually called *speech prostheses* because they play an important role in improving the speech of a child with a cleft palate. There are two major types—a speech bulb, or obturator, and a palatal lift.

A speech bulb, shown in Figure 15, is held in the mouth by a section that covers part of the hard palate and by clasps that attach to the teeth. The bulb itself is a piece of plastic designed to fit the shape of the throat but somewhat smaller so that the child can breathe through the nose with the bulb in place. This prosthesis functions by filling in the space in the throat so that the throat walls have to move only a short distance to completely close off the nose from the mouth during speech.

A palatal lift helps to achieve closure by a different method. The lift, which also covers the hard palate and attaches to the teeth, includes a thin tail-piece of plastic that lifts the soft palate up and back to a position where it can

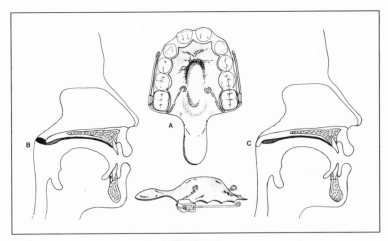

FIGURE 15
The use of speech prostheses to improve closure. Both the speech bulb
(left) and the palatal lift (right) can be used to close off the nose from the
mouth. A speech bulb is held in the mouth by a section that covers the hard
palate and by clasps that attach to the teeth (A). When it is in place (B), the
bulb fills most of the space at the back of the throat so that the closure is
easier to achieve. A palatal lift aids closure by lifting the soft palate so that it
comes in contact with the back of the throat (C).

make contact with the back throat wall (Figure 15). As with
the speech bulb and pharyngeal flap surgery, closure can
then be completed by the side walls of the throat moving in.

As mentioned earlier, both the palatal lift and the speech
bulb can be used permanently or temporarily as training devices to improve speech. This second use will be described in
detail in Chapter 7.

In this chapter we have described some of the ways in
which clefts are treated by surgery. Our descriptions have
been general, and you will probably want to obtain more de-
tailed information to understand fully the treatment your
child will receive and to make necessary decisions. Your sur-

geon and the other specialists on the cleft palate team are the best sources of this information. The material presented here should make it easier for you to ask questions and learn what you need to know.

Chapter 4
FEEDING A CHILD WITH A CLEFT

Feeding certainly is an early concern for the parents of a child with a cleft lip or palate. One of your first questions after the birth of your child may have been, "Will I have problems feeding the baby?"

There is no simple answer to this question. Some children and parents experience no difficulties in feeding, while others have quite significant problems. However, even if there are problems, you may be sure of one thing: your child's nutritional needs can be met. It goes without saying that good nutrition is of utmost importance for a child's satisfactory growth and development. Good nutrition and the health it promotes are also needed to fight off infections and encourage healing following surgical repair of the lip and palate. Therefore, it is important to see your primary-care doctor on a regular basis to make sure your child is getting the nourishment he or she needs for normal development.

Feeding problems in children with clefts vary from baby to baby, just as they do in children having normal mouth structures. They also vary with the extent of the cleft. Children with clefts of the hard and soft palate often have the most severe problems, particularly with sucking. Normal vigorous sucking requires a seal and closure between the nose and mouth. Because a cleft of the hard and soft palate reduces pressure buildup in the mouth, sucking is considerably weaker. If the cleft involves just the lip or just a small portion of the soft palate and uvula, sucking behavior may be affected only slightly.

Problems with sucking make it difficult for a child to get formula or milk to the back part of the mouth, where reflexive swallowing occurs. Our job is to help the child accomplish this. Children with clefts, like all infants, possess the innate reflex to suck, and they will try to do so. In feeding, we want to minimize the frustration and fatigue involved in not being able to suck effectively. Even if it is ineffective, sucking activity should be encouraged since these actions appear to be important in oral and palatal development and in the development of speech.

Methods of Feeding Liquids

The possibility of breastfeeding a child with a cleft palate should not be ruled out, but it will not be easy. The success of breastfeeding usually depends on the extent of the cleft. If the baby can create a seal between the breast and the mouth structure, satisfactory suction may be possible. A very small number of mothers have been successful with breastfeeding.

The majority of parents and caretakers feed children with clefts from bottles. Many types of bottles and nipples are available. Sometimes specially designed ones are used for babies with clefts. It is also possible to modify regular bottles and nipples for such use. The bottle most frequently recommended is made of soft plastic that can be squeezed gently to assist the baby's sucking. A soft nipple with an enlarged opening can help to increase the flow of milk. The opening in a regular nipple can be enlarged by making slits or cross-cuts with a razor blade. Your doctor or pediatric nurse will advise you in choosing a bottle and nipple that is best for your baby's needs.

During feeding, your baby should be held in a semi-sitting or upright position to take advantage of gravity during swallowing. This position minimizes the loss of liquids directly into the nose and reduces the possibility of choking or gagging. In spite of such precautions, some liquids and foods will get into the baby's nose before the palate is repaired. This should cause no significant problems and will probably happen less often as your child learns how to direct food to the back part of the mouth.

Burping is an important part of feeding any child, and babies with clefts usually require more frequent burping because they tend to swallow more air than other children.

Feeding a child with a cleft may take longer than feeding other children, but this too will improve with time. If your baby falls asleep before a sufficient amount of formula is taken, it might be advisable to plan more frequent feedings of smaller amounts. It is important to make sure that neither you nor your child becomes over-tired during feeding.

In solving problems related to feeding, experimentation is the rule. Methods that are comfortable, enjoyable, and successful for others may not work for you and your baby. Keep trying until you find what works best for you. In the meantime, the best general advice we can offer is to have patience and confidence.

Chris McNamara finally learned how to feed her baby daughter, Tammy, after trying a lot of different things and going through some pretty rough times. At first, Chris wanted to breastfeed Tammy, but she quickly discovered that the baby, who was born with a cleft of her hard and soft palate, just could not get enough milk. Even bottlefeeding was difficult, and both mother and child became very frustrated by all the hard work it took to get just a little formula into Tammy's stomach.

But Chris and Tammy kept trying, and Chris got helpful advice from the other parents in her cleft palate support group. Many of them had problems feeding their children, and when talking with them, Chris realized she wasn't alone. With the help of their suggestions and the advice of the cleft palate team, Chris finally worked out a feeding system that suited both her and her daughter. She found just the right kind of soft plastic bottle and soft nipple, and fed

Tammy small amounts of formula every three hours. At six months, Tammy weighed just what she should for her age and size. She had a healthy appetite and could hardly wait to get her gums into some solid foods.

Weaning and Feeding Solid Foods

Like Tammy, your child will probably begin eating some solid food at about six months of age. Your doctors will advise you about the best time to introduce solids and also to wean your baby from the bottle. Weaning is often done at the time that the hard and soft palates are surgically repaired.

The first solids introduced into your child's diet will be small amounts of strained foods. At the beginning, it may be helpful to dilute or liquify the food, but it should be fed by spoon and not by bottle. As your child gets used to eating from a spoon, the amounts and varieties may be increased, depending on the child's appetite and acceptance. Adding new foods one at time is always a good idea since some foods can cause allergic reactions in children. If there is a reaction to a particular food, be sure to report it to your doctor.

New foods with different tastes and textures may not initially be accepted by your child, but with patient encouragement, he or she will eventually learn to enjoy many kinds. When feeding a child with an unrepaired cleft, it is wise to avoid spicy or acidic foods such as citrus fruit juices because they can irritate the tender nasal tissues.

Proper feeding of any child takes time, and feeding a child with a cleft palate requires more than the average quota of a parent's time and patience. When making the change to solid foods, feeding small portions slowly is usually the best approach. Five or six small feedings a day may be preferable and more enjoyable than three larger meals. No matter what your schedule, never force-feed your child. Children will eat when they are hungry.

Drinking from a cup is usually encouraged at about eight to ten months of age. Your doctor or surgeon may have specific suggestions about the scheduling of this change. Generally, by the time the palate is repaired, the child has already been weaned from the bottle and is taking liquids by cup and eating with a spoon.

Feeding After Surgery

Immediately following surgical repair of the hard and soft palate, the child will be fed by putting a solution directly into the bloodstream through a needle in the veins. Intravenous feeding will probably be done for the first 24 hours after the operation. Then liquids and soft foods will gradually be reintroduced until there has been sufficient healing to resume the diet eaten before surgery. During the healing period, it is not advisable to feed your child hard foods such as cookies, crackers, and toast, which might damage the surgical repair. For the same reason, the child should not be allowed to put hard objects into his or her mouth.

When the palate is completely healed, your child should have adequate separation between the nose and the mouth. The soft palate should also seal off the nasal area during swallowing. These improvements should make eating much easier for both child and parents.

While possible early problems in feeding a child with cleft palate cannot be ignored, they are not unmanageable. Help is available from the cleft palate team, from parent support groups, and from professional organizations that specialize in treating persons with cleft palate. Some of these organizations are listed at the end of this book. In solving your particular problems, don't hesitate to ask questions and to share your concerns. Whatever method of feeding is successful for you and your child, we hope that it results in a close and pleasurable experience.

Chapter 5
EAR PROBLEMS: WHY THEY HAP-PEN AND WHAT CAN BE DONE ABOUT THEM

Earaches and other problems with the ears can be painful, and almost all children are bothered with them at some time. Unfortunately, children with clefts have more than their share. In this chapter, we will identify these problems, describe how they develop, and discuss how they can be treated. First, let's take a quick look at the human ear and the way it works.

The Structure of the Ear

The human ear is divided into three sections (Figure 16). The outer ear is the part that we can see and that we usually refer to when we talk about our ears. This section of the ear is made up of the auricle and the ear canal.

Many of the working parts of the ear are in the middle section. The middle ear is separated from the outer ear by a membrane known as the eardrum. Within the middle ear is a set of connected bones called the ossicles. The ossicles are attached to the inside of the eardrum and to another piece of membrane, the oval window, which separates the middle ear from the inner ear. The middle ear also has an opening at the bottom, the eustachian tube, which connects to the upper part of the back of the throat, above the soft palate.

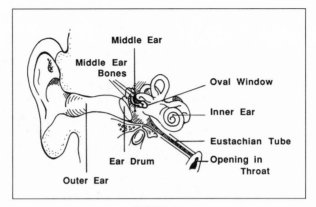

FIGURE 16
The parts of the human ear. The ear drum separates the outer ear from the middle ear. Connected to the ear drum are the ossicles, three small bones that communicate vibrations to the inner ear through the oval window. The eustachian tube connects the middle ear to the throat.

Normally the eustachian tube is collapsed or closed, but it can be opened by muscles in the throat and palate. The tube opens when we swallow, yawn, or blow our noses. This allows air to move between the middle ear and the throat, keeping the middle ear well ventilated and equalizing air pressure on either side of the eardrum. The eustachian tube is opened when we swallow, but the elevation of the soft palate closes it off from the mouth, thus preventing food from getting into the middle ear when eating.

The inner ear is enclosed in a cavity in our skull. It is a complex system of passageways and chambers containing fluids and nerve endings. The nerve endings in the inner ear send messages to the brain, making hearing possible.

This is how the whole system works. A human voice or any other sound causes molecules of the surrounding air to vibrate. These vibrations move down a listener's auditory canal until they come into contact with the eardrum, causing it to vibrate. The vibration of the eardrum is communicated to the tiny bones in the middle ear, which in turn cause the oval window between the middle and inner ear to vibrate. The movement of the oval window sets off vibrations in the fluids in the inner ear, which stimulate the nerve endings in the inner ear. Messages sent to the brain by the nerve endings are heard as sounds.

The human sense of hearing depends on a complex system of many parts that works well for most people most of the time. However, ear problems can develop, and they can have some unpleasant consequences.

Problems in the Middle Ear

Children with clefts have the same kinds of ear problems as other youngsters, but they seem to have them more frequently and often more severely. Problems with the middle ear are the most common among children with clefts. Approximately 38 percent of all children will have had at least one middle-ear infection by the age of three. Although comparable information is not available on children with clefts, a conservative estimate would be that at least 80 percent of them will have had one or more of these conditions by age three.

One middle-ear problem that is particularly bothersome to children with clefts is *otitis media*. This is a medical term describing a condition in which the tissue of the middle ear is inflamed—red, swollen, and hot. There are several possible causes for this condition. The eustachian tube is not working properly; the middle-ear tissue is infected; the child has an allergy.

Otitis media can be painful, but if the child has it for a relatively short period of time—one or two weeks—it usually does not have serious effects. The child's hearing may not be affected, and even if there is a hearing difficulty, it will usually be mild.

Chronic otitis media, however, lasts for a longer time and may present a more serious problem. For example, it may affect the eustachian tube so that air is prevented from getting into the middle ear. This lack of air can cause the eardrum to be stretched, affecting the child's hearing. Improper functioning of the eustachian tube can also prevent the drainage of fluids that develop in the middle ear. A buildup of fluids may affect the function of the eardrum and the ossicles, leading to further hearing problems. If the fluid pressure becomes too great, it may cause a perforation—a hole—in the eardrum. All of these conditions may cause severe pain and are a source of potential damage.

We do not understand fully why a child with a cleft is particularly susceptible to such problems. The most likely cause is difficulty opening the eustachian tubes and allowing air to get into the middle ear. Some of the muscles that do this are attached to the palate, and the cleft may prevent them from functioning properly. It is also possible that a cleft makes it easier for infectious agents such as bacteria and viruses to get into the eustachian tubes and cause inflammation of the tissue. Both these factors may play a role in making children with clefts susceptible to middle-ear problems.

That's the bad news. The good news is that these problems can be treated successfully, especially if they are identified early. It is also good to know that proper care will reduce the possibility that the problems will reoccur. Finally, most children will become less susceptible to otitis media as they grow older.

Treatment of Middle-Ear Problems

Specific treatment programs will differ from one child to the next, since they depend on an assessment of your child's particular problem and his or her stage of development. Several treatments are generally used for otitis media. For example, if your doctor believes that some type of medication will reduce a middle-ear infection or an allergic reaction, this will be the treatment of choice. If the physician is concerned about the amount of fluid in the middle ear, he or she may choose to reduce it by doing a *myringotomy*. This procedure involves inserting a small needle through the eardrum and extracting excess fluids. By reducing the fluid, the ear may return to its normal function.

When middle-ear problems are of long standing or particularly bothersome, physicians often perform a minor surgical procedure in which they create a small opening in the eardrum and insert a tube. This tube, known as a *ventilation tube*, is designed to maintain the opening for an extended period of time, several weeks or months. While it is in place, it relieves pressure and allows air to circulate in the middle ear, making it easier for the ear tissue to return to its normal healthy condition. A ventilation tube also prevents the development of additional ear problems.

Mary Polanski, age four, had a history of middle-ear problems. Her early episodes of ear inflammation had been treated successfully with an antibiotic, but now the treatment was proving ineffective. Mary's otolaryngologist recommended that ventilation tubes be placed in her ears. Mary's mother, Ellen, was concerned about having this surgery done now because Mary was already scheduled for some secondary lip surgery next month. The otolaryngologist called Mary's surgeon and arranged to have both procedures done when Mary was under general anesthesia.

The operation was performed early in June, and Mary came out of it not only with an improved appearance but also with tubes in both her ears. She was soon ready to resume her normal routine, which included playing in her wading pool during the hot days of midsummer. Ellen knew that getting water in the ventilation tubes could irritate the tissue in the middle ear, however, and she asked the otolaryngologist for advice. He referred her to a clinic where she could get ear plugs made for Mary. The summer continued to be hot, and Mary spent a lot of time in her pool. She learned to put her ear plugs in before splashing in the water, and her ears remained healthy.

Because a ventilation tube is always open, water can get into the middle ear when the child is playing in a wading pool, swimming, or washing. The care needed to avoid problems with ventilation tubes is not complicated, but many children, unlike Mary, find it difficult or bothersome. They may have to be reminded to keep water out of their ears and to take other necessary precautions.

Identifying Ear Problems

As we have noted, early detection of ear problems makes them easier to treat. Because it's impractical to have a physician check a child's ears once a week or even once a month, it is important that parents be able to recognize the early signs of possible trouble.

In the first months of life, it is difficult for parents to know whether hearing is normal and whether their child is experiencing ear problems. However, there may be some clues in the child's behavior. Constant crying or frequent rubbing or pulling of the ears, for example, may indicate pain or discomfort caused by middle-ear problems. If you see wet or dried fluid, including blood, in the ear canal, you should suspect that something is wrong with your child's ears. Any or all of these conditions should prompt an early visit to your physician.

Sometimes a child's ear problems will not cause pain but will affect normal hearing. There are ways to recognize this kind of hearing loss in very young children. In play with infants, adults often use sounds as a means of communication. Parents and other adults make cooing noises in an attempt to encourage a baby to coo and gurgle in response. Sometimes we talk to an infant and watch to see if he or she is aware of our presence. Noise-making toys are also used to get a child's attention. All of these activities are normal and healthy and probably contribute to the infant's social and intellectual growth. If your child does not participate in play activities or make noises in response, it may be a sign that she or he is having difficulty hearing. This is something that should definitely be checked by a physician.

John and Sally Bird knew that their six-month-old son Billy, who had a cleft palate, might develop problems with his hearing. Their doctor advised them to observe Billy closely and try to find out if he heard the sounds around him. The Birds noted that when John was playing with the baby and Sally called from the next room, Billy would stop his activities and appear to listen. They decided to put their observations to a test. While John amused Billy with a toy animal, Sally moved quietly to a place where her son couldn't see her and then called out his name very softly. John watched carefully and noticed that Billy responded just about every time his mother called his name.

The Birds decided to check Billy's hearing by doing this little experiment twice a week and noting Billy's response on a calendar. One day about a month after starting the tests, there was no response: Billy did not seem to hear his mother's call. They did the experiment for the next three days, and each time, Billy did not respond to Sally's soft voice, although he seemed to hear if she spoke loudly. When Billy was tested by a hearing specialist, he was found to have a mild hearing loss in both ears. An examination by the otolaryngologist revealed that there was fluid in his ears. Medication was prescribed, and Billy's ears (and hearing) returned to normal in two weeks.

At this point, we would like to re-emphasize that middle-ear problems do not result in a complete loss of hearing. In fact, children with severe problems of this kind can still hear their own voices and usually those of adults who are close by and who talk at normal conversational levels. They often have difficulty, however, hearing soft sounds and sounds produced at a great distance from their ears. For example, such children may not hear a car pulling up in the driveway, a dog barking next door, or someone talking in the next room. They may also have difficulty hearing people in the same room who speak softly or whisper.

As your child grows older, it will be a littler easier to determine if an ear problem is present. A child of three or four can usually tell us about ear pain or hearing difficulties. However, we can't always rely on a child's awareness of a slight loss in hearing, especially if it's not accompanied by ear pain. We must look for signs that suggest a hearing problem. Does the child always turn the television sound to a level higher than that used by other members of the family? Does your daughter or son fail to respond to questions or requests by someone in another room? Does the child avoid or ignore group discussions, particularly when they take place in noisy surroundings? This kind of behavior may suggest the existence of a hearing loss.

At this point, most parents are no doubt saying, "Hold it, this behavior is typical of all children, whether or not they have ear problems." Of course, you're right, but the difference is that children with normal hearing don't *always* respond or behave in the ways described. If they can hear and if it is to their advantage to do so, they respond appropriately. The child with a hearing loss doesn't respond even when it is to his or her advantage. In general, the rule of thumb should be, "If there's a significant lack of response, have the child's hearing checked."

The specialist who will do this job is the audiologist, a professional concerned with identifying and evaluating hearing problems and treating people with such problems. Audiologists can be found in many places. Sometimes they have their own offices, or they may work with an otolaryngologist. They are also affiliated with hospitals, schools, and rehabilitation centers.

When your child is young, you may see an audiologist once or twice a year, usually at the same time you see your ear doctor. The audiologist will ask questions about the child's growth and about your observations of his or her hearing. Then some type of hearing test will be given. When four-year-old Joel Shapiro had his hearing testing, he was placed in a sound-controlled room wearing earphones. Sounds of known loudness and pitch were sent through the

Many professionals are involved in the diagnosis, evaluation, and treatment of cleft lip and palate. Parents and other family members also have an important part to play in the treatment of children with this defect. The following series of photographs, taken at a Cleft Palate Clinic, shows several young patients and their families working with the specialists on the interdisciplinary cleft palate team.

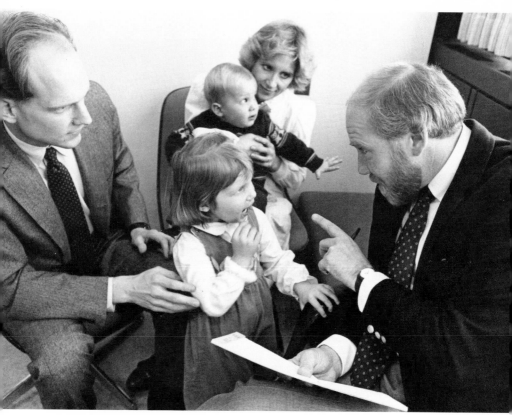

The Gill family has two members with clefts: four-year-old Kristen and two-year-old Brian. When the Gills visited the Cleft Palate Clinic in January, the whole family met with Dr. Karlind Moller, the coordinator of the interdisciplinary team, to discuss plans for Kristen's treatment.

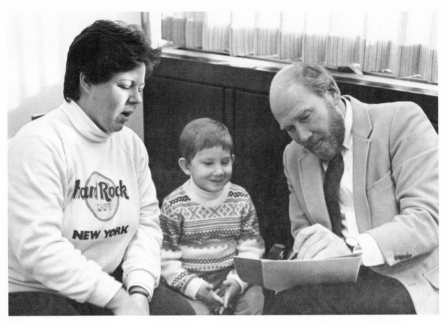

Dr. Moller uses a drawing to help another young patient, five-year-old Trevor Alt, and his mother understand the procedures to be used during Trevor's treatment.

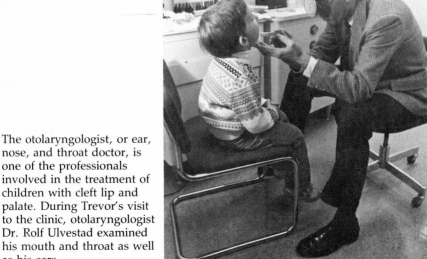

The otolaryngologist, or ear, nose, and throat doctor, is one of the professionals involved in the treatment of children with cleft lip and palate. During Trevor's visit to the clinic, otolaryngologist Dr. Rolf Ulvestad examined his mouth and throat as well as his ears.

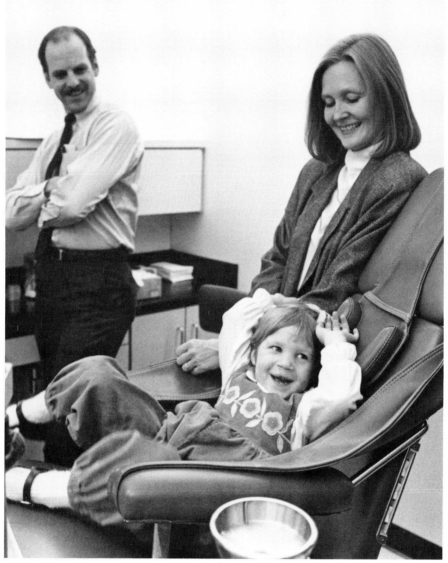

Kristen Gill shares a moment of relaxation with two surgeons on the interdisciplinary team, Dr. Marie Christensen (right), a plastic surgeon, and Dr. Dan Gatto (left), whose speciality is oral surgery.

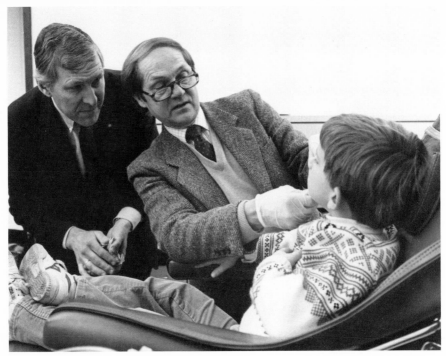

Trevor was examined by an orthodontist, Dr. Gary Carlson (left), and an oral surgeon, Dr. Bill Frantzich (right). These specialists wanted to find out how Trevor's teeth and jaws were developing and how the teeth in the upper and lower jaws came together.

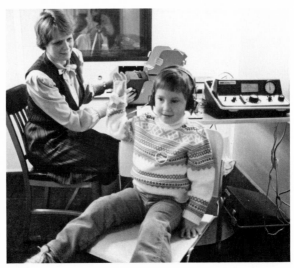

Working in a sound-proof room, Jane Carlstrom, an audiologist, checks Trevor's hearing. If she discovers that he has a hearing loss, she will share her findings with the otolaryngologist, Dr. Ulvestad.

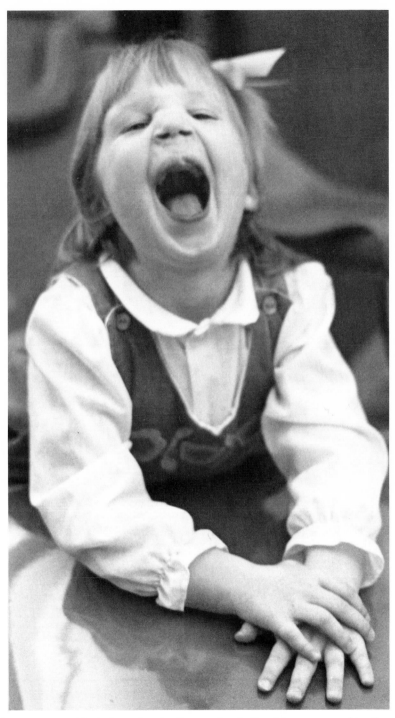

Kristen opens wide to have her teeth examined. Good home care of teeth and regular visits to the dentist are essential in the treatment of a child with a cleft.

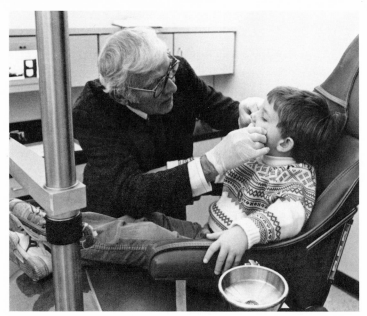

Dr. George Geist, a prosthodontist, takes a good look at Trevor's teeth. This specialist is concerned with the bite of the teeth, the replacement of missing teeth, and, if necessary, the fitting of speech prostheses.

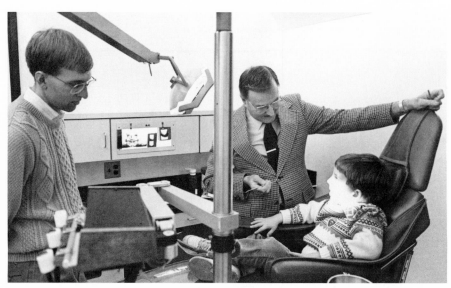

Dr. Kenneth Erickson, a family dentist, talks to Trevor before he looks at his teeth and examines his oral health. The x-rays of Trevor's teeth help make the dental exams more complete. Dr. Ron Grothe, a pediatric dentistry resident, looks on and is learning about the clinic's procedures and interdisciplinary care.

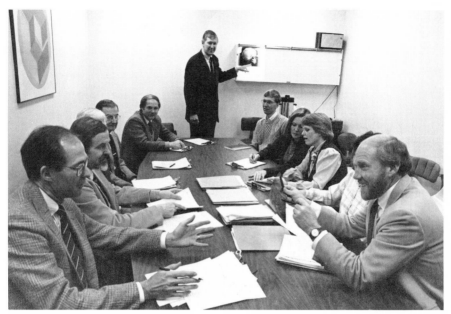

All the specialists on the interdisciplinary team meet to discuss the results of tests on one of their patients and to make recommendations about treatment. Dr. Carlson is pointing out the development of the child's teeth and jaws, shown in an X-ray of the side of the head.

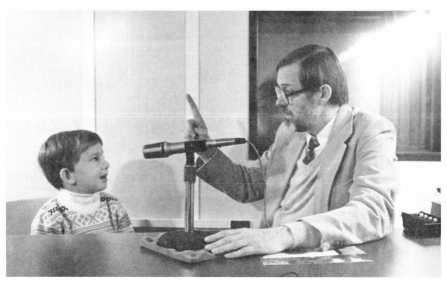

An assessment of speech and language is an important part of the interdisciplinary evaluation. Here a speech clinician, Dr. Clark Starr, is testing Trevor's speech in a sound-proof room. Dr. Starr asks Trevor to say certain sounds, words, and sentences to see how well he is using his mouth parts to produce speech.

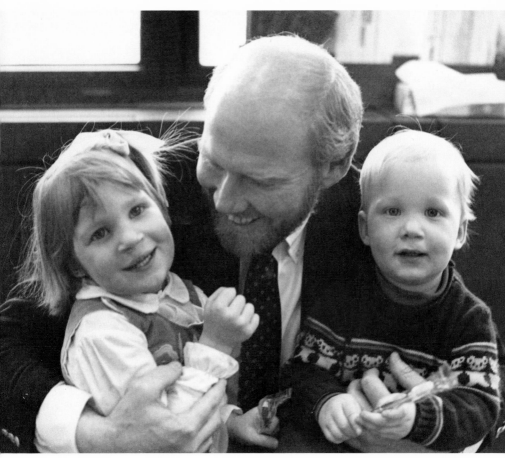

After a long day at the Cleft Palate Clinic, Kristen and Brian Gill say good-bye to their friend Dr. Moller. They will see him again in about one year, when they come in for their next evaluation.

earphones, and the audiologist observed Joel's responses. From these observations, the audiologist concluded that Joel had a slight hearing loss in his left ear. She reported her finding to the otolaryngologist, who then examined Joel to try to find out if his hearing loss was due to an ear problem.

The audiologist's findings are also used in deciding if children like Joel need special assistance so that hearing problems do not interfere with future development of speech and language. If your child is found to need special help, the audiologist will advise you about what aid is required and what role you as parents can play in providing it. If it is appropriate, the audiologist will talk with day-care or nursery-school workers who deal with your child. When your son or daughter reaches school age, an audiologist connected with the school will make tests on a regular basis to identify problems and to guide you and the school staff in meeting your youngster's special needs.

When Melissa Andrews entered kindergarten, her parents talked to the teacher and told her of Melissa's recurrent ear problems. The teacher consulted the school audiologist, who reviewed the child's hearing and speech history and tested her hearing. The audiologist found no hearing loss, but scheduled Melissa for another test in four weeks. She also asked the teacher and Melissa's parents to call her if they noticed any problems.

At the next hearing test, the audiologist discovered that Melissa had developed a mild to moderate hearing loss probably resulting from a middle-ear inflammation. She informed Melissa's parents, who made an appointment with their otolarnygologist, and she also talked to the kindergarten teacher. She suggested that Melissa be seated close to the front of the room during general classroom activities and that the teacher observe her carefully to be certain that she heard instructions. She also suggested it would be helpful if the teacher talked to Melissa for a few moments every day to find out if she was having any problems hearing during special classroom activities or at play with the other children.

With the audiologist's guidance and the teacher's skillful handling of the situation, Melissa experienced no real problems at school. Within a few weeks, ventilation tubes were placed in her ears and her hearing returned to normal.

Ear Problems in Perspective

There are several important things to remember about ear problems of children with clefts. First, such children tend to have problems with their ears and sometimes experience mild to moderate hearing losses. Second, with early identification and proper care, most of the problems can be successfully treated. Third, your careful observation of your child's behavior is extremely useful in identifying ear problems early. Fourth, an audiologist will provide professional help in identifying hearing problems and in providing the special services your child might need. Fifth (and most important in the long run), by the time your child has become a teen-ager, ear problems will usually no longer be a problem.

Chapter 6
CLEFTS AND THE DEVELOPMENT OF TEETH

Many children with clefts can be expected to have some problems with the development of their teeth and jaws. To understand how clefts can affect these parts of the mouth, it is necessary to know something about the structure of the jaws and normal teeth.

The Structure of the Jaws and the Development of Teeth

The bony upper jaw, or maxilla, is the area affected by clefting. If you will look at Figure 17, you will see that the maxilla has three main parts—a central triangular portion (the premaxilla) and a section on each side (the lateral maxillary segments). The lines in the drawing show where these three parts normally fuse or join during a child's development in the womb. Clefts occur along these lines when the normal prenatal fusion does not take place.

The portion of the bony upper jaw that contains the teeth is known as the *alveolar process*, or *alveolar ridge*. At birth, there are usually no visible teeth in this bony ridge, but teeth have been developing deep inside the jaw for some time. As the infant grows, they begin to appear, first the upper and lower front teeth. By the time the child is about two and a half to three years old, he or she usually has a complete set of

55

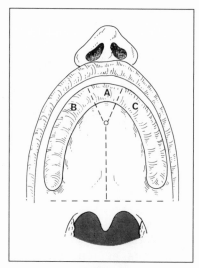

FIGURE 17
Parts of the bony upper jaw. The bony upper jaw is made up of the premaxilla (A) and two lateral maxillary segments (B,C).

primary teeth. These teeth are also known as *deciduous teeth*
because, like the leaves on deciduous trees, they are des-
tined to be shed.

Figure 18 shows the normal number and the names of the
deciduous teeth. You can see from the drawing that the premaxilla of the upper jaw contains the central and lateral incisors. The other upper teeth are in the lateral maxillary segments.

Teeth, of course, are used for chewing, and it is the movable lower jaw, called the *mandible*, that makes this action
possible. As the mandible closes, the teeth of both jaws come
into contact. This contact is known as the bite or *occlusion*. (A
side view of the normal occlusion of the deciduous teeth is
shown in Figure 19.)

The shape of the lower dental arch is about the same as
that of the upper arch so that the teeth can touch each other
in occlusion. However, as you can see in the drawing, the

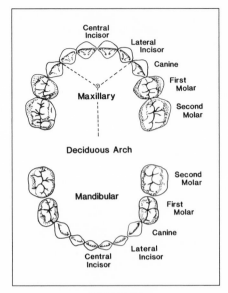

FIGURE 18
The deciduous teeth.

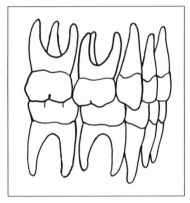

FIGURE 19
The occlusion or bite of the deciduous teeth.

front teeth in the upper jaw are slightly in front of and over-lap the teeth in the lower jaw. These positions are referred to as *normal overjet* and *overbite*. The function of the sharper

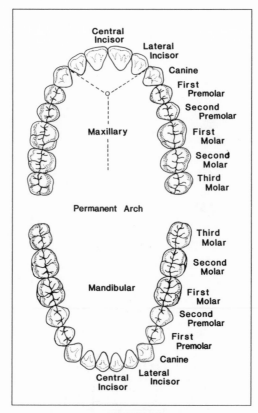

FIGURE 20
The permanent teeth.

front teeth is to bite off and tear food. The back teeth, which serve to grind and chew food, contact each other, biting surface to biting surface.

As a child grows, the deciduous teeth are gradually lost, and the permanent or secondary teeth erupt into the dental arches. Generally, the deciduous teeth are lost in the same sequence in which they appeared, the front teeth before the back teeth. The age at which this change takes place varies from child to child. Generally, the deciduous incisor teeth start to fall out at about six to eight years, and the canines

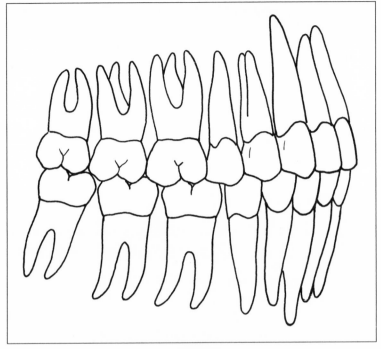

FIGURE 21
The occlusion of the permanent teeth.

and molars are lost from about nine to twelve years. During this same period, the permanent teeth are erupting, again in a sequence from front to back. The phase during which some deciduous teeth and some permanent teeth are present is called the *mixed dentition phase.*

Many of the permanent teeth have the same names and positions as the deciduous teeth, as you can see in Figure 20. However, there are several more permanent teeth: the premolars, or first and second bicuspids, and the third molars, or wisdom teeth. As with the deciduous teeth, the four upper incisors are in the premaxillary segment of the the jaw.

Figure 21 shows the occlusion of the permanent teeth from the side. As with primary teeth, normal overjet and overbite exist in the relationship between the front teeth in the upper and lower jaws. Upper and lower arch forms are still similar, but the upper jaw is slightly longer and wider. In many ways, the upper dental arch is shaped something like a cover over the lower arch.

With time, the upper and lower jaws, as well as the entire face, continue to grow and develop in a somewhat downward and forward direction. The normal upper jaw has achieved almost all of its side-to-side growth by the time a child is approximately five or six years old, but up-and-down growth continues until early adolescence. The mandible (lower jaw) may not reach its full size until sixteen to eighteen years of age.

These general growth patterns may be somewhat different from child to child and are, of course, influenced by inherited characteristics of facial size and shape. The important thing to remember is that growth and development of the teeth, jaws, and face take place over time. This information will help you to understand when certain treatments for a child with cleft palate are most appropriate and most effective.

The Effects of Clefts on Teeth and Bite

Clefts have different effects on the teeth depending on their location and size. The teeth of a child born with only a cleft lip, for example, will probably be no different from those of a child without this defect. This also may be true for a child with an incomplete or even complete cleft of the secondary palate or one occurring just in the roof of the mouth. As long as the alveolar process of the upper jaw is not involved, the number and generally the position of the teeth are not affected. If the cleft *does* involve this area of the jaw, however, we can expect some differences in the teeth. It is important to know that, even in this situation, there will be more similarities to the normal pattern than there will be differences.

It is easy to see why a cleft of the bony alveolar ridge can significantly affect development of teeth. The separation, either on one side or both, typically goes all the way through the ridge to the floor of the nose. In most cases, the early surgery that repaired the lip and palate did not include the cleft in the alveolar ridge. As we have explained, surgical repair of a cleft in this area is usually done at a later date, when the upper jaw has grown more.

A cleft in the alveolar ridge has two different effects on the jaw segments and teeth. One is caused by the separation that exists between the sections of the bony upper jaw, along the normal fusion lines. If the cleft is bilateral (on both sides), the premaxilla is separated from both of the lateral maxillary segments. In this situation, the only bony attachment that the premaxilla has is with the vertical bony partition of the nose, the septum. With lack of fusion on both sides, the premaxilla and the lateral maxillary segments are subject to movement. If the cleft involves only one side of the alveolar ridge, the lateral maxillary segment on that side may be movable (Figure 22).

Forces or pressures acting on these jaw segments over time can cause them to change position because they lack bony connection. A force pushing the movable segments out is the tongue. The cheeks and lip, on the other hand, push the movable segments in. Since the tongue is not involved in clefting, the outward force exerted would be similar to that in a person without a cleft. Surgical closure of a cleft in the lip, however, exerts an inward force on the segments that may cause them to be somewhat displaced. This is called *arch collapse* and results in a condition commonly known as *crossbite*.

Bilateral crossbite occurs when the upper teeth in the movable segments are positioned inside the lower teeth, in the direction of the tongue. Arch collapse and crossbite may also result from a unilateral cleft, but then only the jaw segment on the cleft side is affected (Figure 23). In either situation, the degree of crossbite is generally mild and can usually be corrected by orthodontic treatment at the appropriate time.

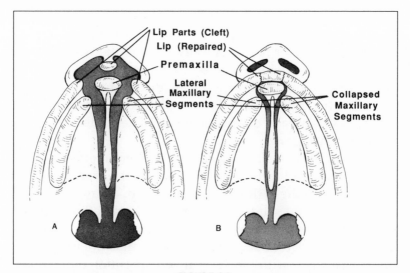

FIGURE 22

Bilateral clefts in the lip and alveolar ridge and displacement of jaw segments following repair of the lip. A bilateral cleft of the upper jaw (A) causes the three jaw segments to be separated from each other. Because the segments lack bony continuity, they may be subject to movement. After the clefts of the lip are repaired, pressure exerted on the segments may cause them to move inward (B). This is known as arch collapse and results in crossbite, a condition in which the teeth in the displaced upper jaw segments are positioned inside the lower teeth.

Arch collapse is one of the major effects of clefts in the alveolar ridge and palate. A cleft in the alveolar ridge can also affect the development and position of individual teeth. Both primary and permanent teeth may be missing, poorly formed, or out of position in and around the region of the cleft. There may also be extra teeth. The teeth most frequently missing or poorly formed are the lateral incisors because they develop closest to the lines of alveolar clefts. Not every person with a cleft will have missing teeth or the other problems mentioned, but they are all possibilities.

Peter Howard, for example, had his own individual set of dental problems. Peter, who was seven, had a unilateral cleft that extended through the alveolar ridge on the right side.

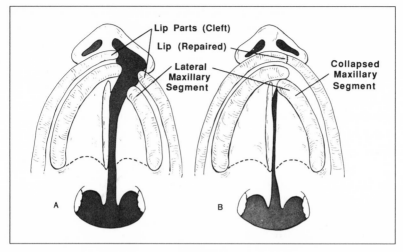

FIGURE 23
Unilateral cleft in the lip and alveolar ridge and displacement of jaw segments following repair of the lip. When the cleft is unilateral (A), only the jaw segment on the side where the cleft is located lacks bony continuity. The pressure exterted by a repaired unilateral cleft lip may cause inward movement of only one jaw segment (B).

His parents were very concerned when they noticed a tooth erupting out of position in the front part of the roof of their son's mouth. Another tooth, the permanent central incisor on the cleft side, was emerging in a rotated, or twisted, position. The worried parents wondered whether such dental problems were unusual in cleft cases and whether anything could be done about them.

The dental specialists on the cleft palate team explained that Peter's situation was not unusual; in fact, it was almost to be expected. The tooth that had erupted into the palate was an extra tooth. Since it was causing no problem, the specialists recommended leaving it there for a while. In fact, they explained to Peter's parents that there was an advantage in not removing it in order to preserve the bone around it. The doctors also told them that the rotated upper front tooth could be straightened in the future but that the timing would depend on how much bone support there was for this tooth. Peter's parents were pleased to learn that X-rays taken of the cleft area showed a developing permanent lateral incisor (the tooth often missing in such situations). Although the lateral incisor was smaller than normal, the specialists thought it would be usable for the long term.

Peter's situation is only one of many that can occur when there is a cleft involving the bony alveolar ridge. As you have seen, such clefts can and often do affect the position of the jaw segments as well as the development and position of individual teeth in the cleft area. Fortunately, these problems are treatable and the results are usually very satisfactory. Like all treatment for cleft lip and palate, however, dental treatment takes time.

Dental Treatment of Children with Clefts

For all children, the basic objectives of dental care are healthy teeth and gums and an occlusion or bite that is satisfactory in both function and appearance. This is just as true for a child with cleft lip or palate as for any other child.

The treatment for healthy teeth and gums is preventive and should be no problem for parents or children. It does take commitment on the part of parents, however, to make sure that regular appointments are made with the dentist and that the home-care program is the best it can be. We strongly recommend that children first see a pediatric dentist or family dentist at approximately eighteen months to two years of age.

Lenore Johnson was very apprehensive about bringing her daughter Kristine to the pediatric dentist for the first time. Kristine was two years old, and her mother knew that she should be started on regular preventive care, including cleaning and fluoride treatment. Lenore's own dental experiences as a child had not been positive. When she and Kristine came for their appointment, Lenore told the dentist how she had hated "drilling for cavities." The dentist pointed out that Kristine had no cavities and that regular professional and home care should prevent her from ever getting any. Kristine's first visit to the dentist was a very positive experience, and she came home proudly wearing a badge signifying membership in the "No Cavities Club." When it was time for her next six-month checkup, she was ready and eager to go.

For children with clefts, healthy teeth and gums make the best foundation for any future dental procedures that may be required. These procedures, which involve several dental specialists, will be planned according to the child's stages of development. This is a very important point to remember. The specialists on the cleft palate team will observe your child's dental and facial development over time and help you make decisions regarding the timing of appropriate treatment.

In addition to your family dentist, the dental specialists most commonly involved in the treatment of cleft palate are the orthodontist, the oral surgeon, and the prosthodontist. Frequently, two or more of these specialists participate in providing treatment so that the best results can be achieved. But let's discuss the concerns of each dental speciality separately.

Orthodontics

The orthodontist is concerned with the position of the teeth in the upper and lower jaws and the occlusion or bite when the teeth come together. The goal of this specialist is that your child have the best possible bite in both function and appearance. To achieve this, the orthodontist may need to reposition individual teeth and the bony segments of the upper jaw with braces on the teeth or other appliances placed in the mouth.

As we have seen, the segments of the upper jaw may move because there is no bony connection between them. Such movement may result in arch collapse and crossbite, in which the upper and lower teeth do not come together in the best way. Crossbite can be corrected orthodontically by moving the bony segments with appliances that fit in the mouth. These appliances vary in design and function, but they all guide the bony segments or teeth into more normal positions. Depending on the severity of the crossbite and the child's stage of development, surgical repositioning in combination with orthodontics may be needed. In some cases of crossbite, only the teeth need to be repositioned rather than the bony segments of the jaw itself. This is usually done with the orthodontic braces commonly used for straightening teeth.

Decisions regarding the most appropriate orthodontic treatment and the best timing for it are made by the orthodontist in consultation with the other dental specialists on the team. These decisions are based on the type and severity of the cleft as well as on the growth and development of your child. Here are some of the times when orthodontic treatment might be considered for a child with a cleft in the bony upper jaw:

1. before the hard palate is closed, in an attempt to position the bony jaw segments more favorably for surgery;

2. when both primary and permanent teeth are present, to position the bony jaw segments more favorably for surgical repair of the alveolar cleft or to align individual teeth for better appearance and function;

3. when the child has his or her permanent teeth, to achieve the final positioning of the bony segments as well as the best alignment of the individual teeth.

In many children with clefts, orthodontic treatment can be postponed until final correction can be done on permanent teeth. It is important to remember that bite and individual tooth position may not be ideal in the primary teeth and mixed primary and permanent teeth phases. Even if this is so, chewing food should be no problem.

Oral Surgery

The particular concern of the oral surgeon is repairing the cleft in the alveolar ridge and correcting jaw deformities that may develop over time. Surgical repair of the alveolar cleft on one side or both is frequently done with a bone graft, taking a piece of bone from the hip and grafting it into the opening in the bony ridge. This procedure offers several advantages:

1. It provides more bone support for the permanent teeth;
2. It provides more stability of the bony segments of the upper jaw;
3. It closes any openings that remain under the lip and extend up into the nose.

The improved bone support for the permanent teeth provided by oral surgery will enable the orthdontist to align individual teeth in the cleft area. The increased stability of the bony segments will give another dental specialist, the prosthodondist, a much better situation in which to construct a bridge replacing any missing teeth.

The most appropriate time to consider repair of the alveolar cleft again depends upon the type and severity of the cleft and the development of individual permanent teeth, as well as upon the general development of the child. The decision for scheduling surgery will be based on the observations and concerns of all the other specialists and the oral surgeon.[9]

In March, Dan Satterly had bone graft surgery to repair the cleft in his alveolar ridge. The tissues healed well, and there was now good bone in the cleft area. In September, seven-year-old Dan started in a new school, and his parents, Paul and Jean, were distressed when he came home crying on the first few days. Dan was having problems with one of his classmates, Sally, who was teasing him about his teeth. Over the summer, Dan's upper central incisor on the cleft side had come in sideways, and, in its rotated position, it looked like a

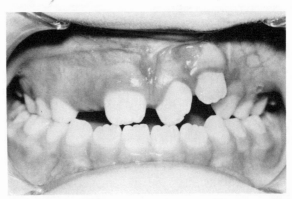

This sequence of photographs shows orthodontic treatment being used to straighten the upper front teeth of a person with a cleft. A. As a result of a cleft in the alveolar ridge, the upper left central incisor is in a rotated position, and the lateral left incisor is erupting out of place.

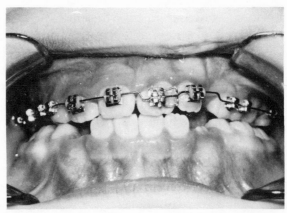

B. After a bone graft to provide more support for the teeth and to allow them to be moved, orthodontic appliances are put in place.

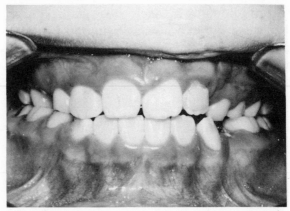

C. After the first phase of orthodontic treatment is completed, the braces are removed. The teeth are now in a much better position. Another phase of orthodontic treatment will be needed later.

sharp knife blade. Sally called Dan "Sabre Tooth" and "Dracula," and her persistent teasing made it difficult for him to adjust to his new school.

When Dan was seen by the interdisciplinary team, it was suggested that the orthodontist begin a phase of treatment to straighten the rotated tooth. This treatment was now possible because there was sufficient bone in the area to move the tooth. Dan's eyes lit up when he found out that his tooth could be straightened—and soon!

During the next few months, braces were used to straighten the rotated tooth and to move Dan's other incisor teeth into better positions. When this phase of treatment was completed, the braces were removed, although Dan and his parents were told that braces would be needed again when more of his permanent teeth had emerged. Dan was proud of his appearance and pleased that he could chew better. He was also much happier at school since Sally had stopped her teasing. (The accompanying sequence of photographs shows Dan's teeth before, during, and after treatment.)

In addition to repairing the alveolar cleft, the second major concern of the oral surgeon is the correction of any jaw deformities that may develop over time. As we mentioned earlier, the bony segments of the upper jaw may require repositioning to obtain the best possible bite. If this cannot be accomplished by orthodontic treatment alone, a surgical assist may be needed.

Surgery to reposition the jaw segments is sometimes required in cases of severe crossbite. In addition to the side-to-side crossbite described earlier, a front-to-back deformity may also become apparent as the child's jaw grows. To correct these problems, the oral surgeon, again in consultation and cooperation with the other dental specialists, may decide to operate to change the position of the jaws. The operation may involve moving forward part or all of the upper jaw; an alternative is moving part or all of the lower jaw backward. As in all surgery on children with clefts, the timing of jaw surgery depends on many individual factors and involves input from several specialists.

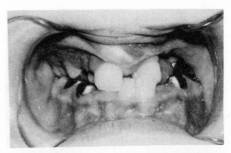

Different Stages in Orthodontic and Prosthodontic Treatment. A. Before orthodontic treatment, several teeth are in crossbite and out of place.

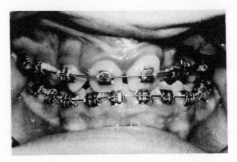

B. During orthodontic treatment, braces are used to correct the crossbite and align the teeth.

Prosthodontics

Like the other dental specialists on the team, the prosthodontist works toward achieving the best dental function and appearance. Replacing missing teeth with a removable partial denture or a fixed bridge is the particular concern of this specialist.

As we have explained, when the cleft involves the alveolar ridge, the permanent lateral incisor is frequently missing on the cleft side of the upper jaw. If the bony segments are stable enough (with or without alveolar bone grafting), the prosthodontist will usually choose to construct a fixed bridge to replace the missing tooth. This is most often done when dental and facial development are complete, at about sixteen to eighteen years of age. In some people, the lateral incisors may be present but poorly formed or underdeveloped. The prosthodontist might consider using crowns to improve the appearance of those teeth.

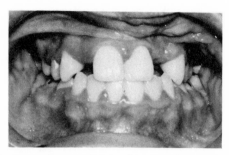

C. After orthodontic treatment, the teeth are in their correct positions, but both upper lateral incisors are missing.

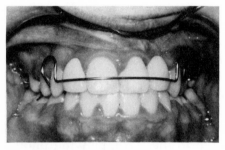

D. A retainer used to reinforce the orthodontic correction also replaces the missing lateral incisors until a fixed bridge is completed.

Replacing a missing tooth or teeth does not have to wait until a fixed bridge can be constructed. Following orthodontic treatment with braces, a retainer is worn for a time to reinforce the orthodontic correction. During this period, an artifical tooth can be added to the retainer until construction of a fixed bridge is appropriate. The accompanying sequence of photographs shows how the prosthodontist used braces to correct the crossbite and align Stephanie Peterson's teeth and how her missing teeth were replaced with artificial ones following treatment.

The prosthodontist may also be involved in treatment relating to speech problems, specifically in fitting and inserting the speech devices described in Chapter 3. Although these devices are temporary, they can significantly improve speech during the time they are worn.

Working Together

Throughout this chapter we have emphasized how the specialists on the cleft-palate team work together to provide the
best dental treatment for a person with a cleft. The case of
John Mackey provides a good illustration.

John was nineteen years old when he was first referred for
interdisciplinary medical and dental evaluation. He had a
cleft lip and palate on the left side, which had been repaired
when he was an infant. A cleft in the alveolar ridge on that
side was unrepaired. Throughout his childhood, John had
received regular dental care, and orthdontic braces had been
placed on his teeth when he was thirteen. His individual
teeth were quite straight and his bite was sufficient for chewing, but he did have some problems with chewing and he
was concerned about the appearance of his teeth. His upper
front teeth did not meet with the lower front teeth, creating
an open bite. John was also missing the upper lateral incisor
on the cleft side. (The condition of John's teeth before treatment are shown in the accompanying photograph.) The X-
rays of the bony cleft revealed that there was not much bone
support for the right central incisor and the right canine
tooth.

The interdisciplinary team decided that the most beneficial
treatment for John would be surgery to close the open bite
between the front jaws and to repair the cleft in the alveolar
ridge with a bone graft. The jaw surgery and some orthodontic treatment would improve his appearance as well improving the bite in the front of his mouth. The bone graft would
have several beneficial results. It would provide better support for the central incisor and canine teeth, stabilize the
bone segments in the upper jaw, and close the opening between the nose and the mouth. Once the surgery was done,
it would be possible for John to have a permanent bridge
made to replace the missing lateral incisor.

Nine months after John Mackey first met with the team, all
the suggested treatments were completed. John's teeth were
greatly improved in appearance and function (as can be seen

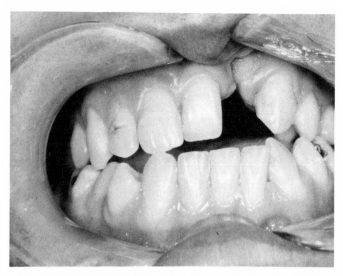

The Results of Surgical, Orthodontic, and Prosthodontic Treatment. A. Before treatment, the cleft in the alveolar ridge is unrepaired. The dental bite or occlusion is also open in front, and the upper left lateral incisor is missing.

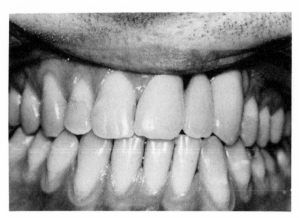

B. After treatment, oral surgery has repaired the cleft, and orthodontic braces have been worn. A fixed bridge has replaced the missing lateral incisor.

in the accompanying photograph), and he was very happy with the results. With regular professional dental care and a good home-care program, he would have a good bite and a great smile for the rest of his life.

Chapter 7
STAYING IN TOUCH: HOW CLEFTS AFFECT SPEECH

At the beginning of this book, we mentioned that cleft palate is a disorder that can be seen, felt, and heard. In this chapter, we will deal with the aspect that can be heard, that is, the problems children with clefts may have with their speech. Before describing these problems, it may be helpful to spend some time explaining what we mean by the term "speech," how speech is produced, and how it is learned.

What Is Speech?

We all know the general meaning of the word "speech." We know what politicians are doing when they make a speech, and we are aware that the speech of a Chinese child sounds different from that of an American child. Linguists, speech clinicians, and others who study speech often use the term in a more limited sense. They think of speech as the individual sounds that humans produce, the way these sounds are combined into words, and the way words are combined into sentences. A brief look at these aspects of speech will make it easier to understand the problems that children with clefts may have in trying to learn how to speak.

First, let's take a look at the way we make the sound we

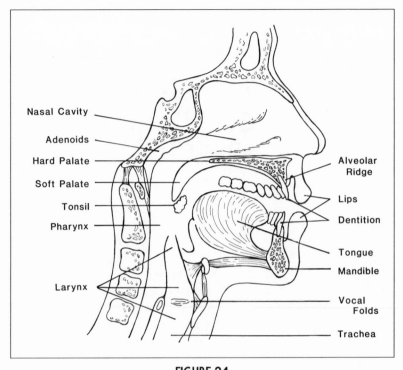

FIGURE 24
The human speech mechanism. Human speech is produced by the functioning of many complex structures in the mouth and throat.

call "voice," that is, the sound we use when we talk, sing, cry, and laugh. This sound is made in our voice box, or larynx (Figure 24). Put your finger on the bump in your throat that is commonly known as the Adam's apple. This is the front wall of your larynx. Now move your fingers down and feel your wind pipe, or trachea. It feels something like a stack of flexible rings. The trachea is a soft pliable tube that runs from your lungs up to your larynx.

Inside the larynx, there are two structures known as vocal folds. They are something like two lips that cover the top of the trachea. When the folds come together, they close off the trachea from the throat and mouth, helping to keep food out of your lungs when you eat.

When your lungs are filled with air, that is, when you have inhaled, the vocal lips can be closed to hold the air inside your lungs. This is what happens when you speak. You fill your lungs with air and close off the trachea with the vocal lips. Then you use the breathing muscles in your chest and abdomen to increase the air pressure in your lungs so that you can force the air through the vocal lips and start them vibrating. When the lips vibrate, they produce sound.

You can change the pitch, loudness, and quality of this sound by changing the breath pressure in your lungs and the length or position of your vocal lips. Try making the sound "ah," as in "saw." Make it loud and then soft. Say it at a high pitch and then at a low pitch. Finally, say "ah" so that it sounds breathy or hoarse. All the differences in sound you have made were accomplished by using your lungs and your vocal lips.

Children with clefts can make the same sounds you have just made. They have normal lungs, tracheas, and larynges. They can produce voice and can control pitch, loudness, and vocal qualities, just as other children do. The problems they have in speaking come from another source.

Vowels

Of course, speech is more than just the ability to produce the sound we call voice. It also includes the individual speech sounds known as vowels and consonants. The vowels we use in English are those that appear in the following words: beat, bit, ate, end, act, past, father, hot, fall, boat, fool, full, above, word. We produce these vowels by making a sound with our larynges and then running the sound through our resonators. Resonators are cavities that change the nature of sound.

The resonators that English speakers use to produce vowels are the mouth and the throat. We make different vowels

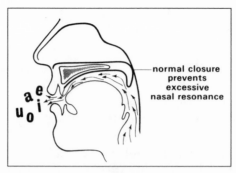

FIGURE 25
Normal closure during vowel production. The raising of the soft palate normally closes off the nose from the mouth and prevents vowels from sound-
ing nasal.

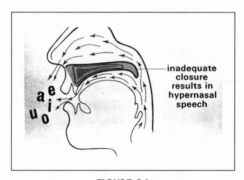

FIGURE 26
Inadequate closure during vowel production. If the soft palate cannot
completely close off the nose from the mouth, nasal-sounding vowels will
be produced.

by changing the size and the shape of these cavities. The eas-
iest way to do this is to change the position of the tongue
within the mouth. Make the sound "ah." Can you sense that
the back of your tongue is low in your mouth? Now try the
sound "ee," as in "see." What happened to your tongue?
You probably raised the front of it. Try a few more vowels
and notice how your tongue moves. These movements
change the resonance characteristics of your mouth and allow you to produce different vowels. If you make the "ah"

sound loud and high in pitch or the "ee" soft and low, the resonators still produce the vowels, but you are using your larynx to change their pitch and loudness.

In addition to the mouth and throat, humans are equipped with another resonator, the nose or nasal cavity. English speakers do not make much use of this resonator in producing vowels, although it plays a very important role in other languages, for example, French. When we are not speaking, the back end of the nose is open and connected with the mouth so that we can breathe through it. When we speak, we close off the nose from the mouth and throat primarily by raising the soft palate (Figure 25). If we fail to raise our palates, the nose becomes a resonator, making our vowels sound nasal (Figure 26).

Try this: Make the vowel "ee." Now try to make it sound nasal, that is, as if the sound is coming through your nose. With a little practice, everyone should be able to do this. If you succeeded in making the vowel sound nasal, this means that you made the sound without raising your palate. Now make several nasal vowels. Listen carefully to the sounds. You can still tell the difference between them, can't you? That is, "ah" sounds like "ah," "ee" like "ee," and so on, whether or not they are nasal.

What all this means to a child with a cleft is that because he or she may have difficulty closing the nose off from the mouth (even after the cleft has been repaired), his or her vowels may sound nasal. These vowels, however, will be recognizable and useful in speech. Furthermore, the child with a cleft can change the pitch and loudness of these vowels in the same manner as a child without a cleft. Unfortunately, there is more to speech than making vowels.

Consonants

Consonants are needed to make speech intelligible. English speakers use the consonants as they appear in these words: pig, big, two, do, cat, go, see, zoo, me, no, shoe, chew, free, very, let, red, thin, then, when, hat, you, garage,

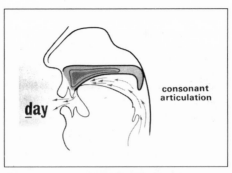

FIGURE 27
Normal closure during the production of consonants. A normal soft palate
closes off the nose from the mouth and allows the build-up of pressure that
is needed for the pronounciation of many consonants.

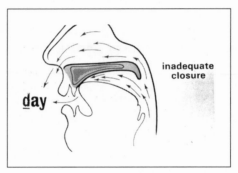

FIGURE 28
Inadequate closure during the production of consonants. When closure is
inadequate because of problems with the soft palate, air escapes through
the nose, and consonants become weak or disappear.

sing. These consonants can be thought of as ways of starting
or stopping the sounds of vowels.

If you put your lips together and start the vowel "ee"with
a little puff of air, you make the word "pea." If you put your
tongue to the gum ridge, behind your upper teeth, and start
the same vowel with a little puff of air, you make the word
"tea." You can do the same thing with the back of your
tongue. If you raise it up so that it touches the back of your
palate and make a little air puff as you begin the "ee," you

make the word "key." Now, try putting your tongue back in the position needed to make the "t" as in "tea." This time, however, let the air leak out slowly instead of in a puff. You will hear a hissing sound that produces the word "see."

There are many things we can do with the tongue and lips to make consonants. Most of these actions, however, depend on the ability to build up some air pressure in the mouth. We need pressure for *t*, *b*, *k*, *s*, and most of the other consonants. To build up pressure in the mouth, it is necessary to raise the soft palate and close off the nose from the mouth and throat (Figure 27). If the palate is not raised, the air pressure that we try to build up will escape out of our noses, and our consonants will disappear or become very weak (Figure 28).

Some consonants are made without closing off the nose. The nose has to be open when we make the consonants *m*, *n*, and *ng* (as in sing). A few other consonants can be made with the nose open or closed. For example, the consonants *h*, *r*, and *l* can be produced either way. When the nose is closed off, they will sound normal; when it's open, they will be recognizable, though they may sound nasal.

At this point, it should be evident that children with cleft palates may have trouble producing some pressure consonants. Because they often have difficulty closing the nose off from their mouth, even after surgical repair of the palate, they may not be able to build up the necessary air pressure in their mouths. Clefts do not prevent these children from placing their lips and tongue in the positions needed to produce the consonants, but they may make it difficult to produce them in a clear and easily understood manner.

What Is Language?

A child must know a great deal more than how to make vowels and consonants in order to speak intelligibly and to understand others. He or she must learn a language, which is a far more difficult task. Fortunately, most children with clefts have all the potential needed for learning a language. They require the same kinds of parental help that other children need, and occasionally a little extra help, but they usually learn to use language as well as their peers.

"Language" is another word that we all understand in a general sense. It refers to the way we combine speech sounds or written letters to produce words, the way we attach meaning to these words, and the way we combine words into phrases and sentences that convey our thoughts and feelings. If you ever had to diagram sentences in a high-school English class or learn a second language, you may be painfully aware of the complexity of language and how difficult it is to learn.

It is almost unbelievable that most children learn to master the complexities of language by the time they are four or five years old. They don't have as big a vocabulary as their parents, but they do know how to make the word "drink" plural by adding "s" and to make it past tense by substituting an "a" for the "i" (drank for drink). They also know how to tell the difference between "drink" as a noun ("I want a drink") or as a verb ("I drink milk") by its use in a sentence. Of course, they make some errors along the way, but they do learn these things at a very early age.

Learning Language

The way in which children learn speech and language continues to perplex linguists, child psychologists, and speech clinicians. At present, we don't know all the details, but we do have some general notions of what is happening when a child learns this vital means of communication.

For example, we know that a child must be exposed to people speaking in order to learn language. We are pretty sure that language and speech learning will take place most efficiently if adults acknowledge, reward, and respond to the child's efforts to produce speech. Precise details about how adults do these things are not clear. It is very clear, however, that millions of parents have done whatever is needed to help their children learn to speak and that most of them did not have to think about doing it. Let's look at some of the things parents do instinctively that seem to be of importance to their children's speech and language development. We'll start with how they expose their children to speech and language.

From birth on, parents talk to children or talk in their presence. Some of this "talk" consists of soft cooing, singing, or humming and saying things like "baby hungry," "baby sleepy," or "pretty baby." Often adults talk to each other about everyday concerns while holding a child or standing near the crib.

Some experts believe it is important for at least some of this talking activitity to take place when the child appears to be enjoying life. For example, they suggest that it is helpful to talk to a child while he or she is being held, being fed, or just waking up, especially if the baby seems to be in good spirits. According to these specialists, it is important that children learn to associate speech with pleasant sensations. Of course, that doesn't mean parents should remain silent when a child is uncomfortable or in pain. Talking at those times may be very beneficial. It does suggest, however, that we should pay special attention to children when they are happy rather than using those moments to concentrate on our own concerns.

At the same time that we are talking to young children, they are beginning to make their own noises. Initially, they coo and goo and produce many other weird and wonderful sounds. It seems obvious that children enjoy making these sounds. Most experts believe it is important that they do make them and that parents respond to a child's efforts, cooing and gooing in return.

Between four and six months, children make sounds in ways that suggest they are gaining control over their speech mechanisms. They are able to produce most of the vowels and consonants that they will eventually use when they start to talk. Of course, they continue to make many sounds that are not part of adult language. Somewhere toward the end of this period, a child may start repeating sounds and syllables. For example, Mark may be heard saying "la-la-la" or "ma-ma-ma" or "kee-kee-kee." This suggests that he is listening to the sounds being made and has sufficient control to repeat them. It also suggests that the process is enjoyable. We call this stage of language development babbling.

During this period, parents continue to talk to their children, and as a child's utterances become clearer, the adults often imitate them. That is, when Peggy says "ga-ga-ga," her parents repeat "ga-ga-ga." The high point of this period takes place when Peggy says "ga-ga," her parents respond "ga-ga," and Peggy answers with another "ga-ga." Here we have real communication with speech. This imitation behavior will grow and expand over several months. During this time, Peggy may be heard making strings of syllables in ways that sound very much like adult speech, even though we don't understand what she is saying.

Somewhere between the ages of twelve and eighteen months, most children will say their first words. The exciting event often happens in this way. Lisa is standing next to the crib and hears baby Sam say "mama." Immediately, she picks the child up, says "mama," and Sam repeats "mama." After this happens two or three times, Lisa may be in another room when she hears "mama," and she will quickly go to the baby's side. Subsequently, she may say to Sam, "Give the spoon to mama," and Sam will hand her the spoon. The ultimate evidence that the meaning of the word is understood comes when Sam's father, Al, picks up the fussing baby, who continues to fuss and call for "mama" until Lisa appears and the fussing stops.

Of course, sometimes the first word is not one that adults use. The very same scenario could take place when Sam says "ee-ee" instead of "mama," if Lisa and Al observe correctly that "ee-ee" means mother.

How does the fact that a child has a cleft palate affect this learning process? In most respects, it will have little effect. Although the cleft palate may not have been repaired during most of this early learning period, the child will make baby noises, including cooing and gooing. She or he will play with these sounds, string syllables together, respond to the parents' encouragement, and eventually learn to say words. During this process, the child will need to hear the parents and other adults talk and have them respond to and reward efforts at speech. In this respect, the child with a cleft may need no more parental attention than children without clefts, but he or she will certainly need as much.

One thing that may differ for children with clefts is that some of their early babbling may sound nasal. The vowels they make will be identifiable but will have a nasal sound. Another difference may be that the consonants these children say may consist primarily of *m, n, k, g, l, r*. Consonants that require pressure in the mouth, such as *p* and *b* or *t* and *d*, may be missing or not clearly produced. These consonants should begin to appear after surgical closure of the palate. First words, however, may appear before a child has mastered those pressure consonants. If this happens, the first words may not sound like the words as they are said by adults.

Karen Olson, who had a cleft palate, was fourteen months old when she started to say words. Her parents, David and Norah, were delighted when Karen learned to say "mama." She had no trouble with this word because "m" is a nasal sound, not a pressure sound. Instead of saying "daddy," however, Karen said something that sounded like "ah-ee" or "nah-nee." At first, both David and Norah were distressed by their daughter's inability to call her father by the familiar name. They felt better, however, after talking to their speech clinician, who explained why Karen had problems with the consonant "d" and why she sometimes substituted the nasal "n" instead.

The speech clinician told Norah and David that Karen would learn correct articulation later and that the crucial point now was that their daughter was beginning to use language to communicate. It was more important that Karen knew what her parents meant when they said "more milk" and that they understood that she wanted more when she said "mo-eekee" than it was for the child to produce an adult version of the word "milk." Once Norah and David understood this, they were able to get on with the process of talking to their daughter and responding to her efforts to speak.

If Karen's parents had noticed that their daughter was not making sounds and not paying attention to the sounds around her, then they would have had reason to be concerned. As we explained earlier, such behavior may be a sign of hearing loss and should be reported to the family physician or audiologist.

Effects of Clefts on Learning Speech and Language: A Summary

It might be helpful at this point to summarize what we have said so far about the way in which children with clefts learn to speak.

1. Babies with cleft palates can make noise and control their pitch and loudness in the same way as other children do.

2. Making these sounds is important for speech development, and parents should encourage their children when they make baby noises.

3. As children grow, they will play with sound, string sounds together, babble, and imitate adults in ways that sound like speech. Again, parents should encourage this activity.

4. When a child begins to use words in a meaningful way, parents should listen carefully and respond.

5. Children with cleft palates that have not been surgically closed will usually pronounce vowels in a nasal manner and will have difficulty producing consonants that require air pressure.

6. Regardless of how their speech sounds, it is important that children with clefts learn to understand and use speech and language. To do this, they will need the encouragement and help of their parents.

One final point: In our discussion so far, we have stressed the importance of the things that parents do to help their children acquire speech and language. For the most part, parents do these things in a very natural way, and they do them whether or not their child has a cleft palate. It is equally natural, however, for parents to be concerned about the speech of a child with a cleft.

There are at least three things that parents can do to deal with these concerns. First, you can do what you are doing right now: read about the subject. Second, you can talk to the speech clinician who works with your cleft-palate team. This specialist in speech and language problems can help you to understand the situation and suggest ways in which you can help your child acquire speech. Third, you can join a support group made up of parents who have children with clefts. Such groups provide an opportunity to learn more about clefting and to share experiences related to raising children with clefts. Your cleft-palate team can help you contact a parent's group in your vicinity.

What Happens To Speech After Surgery?

Most children with cleft palates will have them surgically closed at about one year of age. After surgery, you can expect some changes in speech. Your son or daughter will sound less nasal and will begin experimenting with those consonants that require air pressure. These changes will not occur overnight but will usually become evident a few months after surgery. In most instances, your child's speech will improve without direct help from anyone. Sometimes, however, the improvement doesn't take place as expected.

If your child's speech hasn't changed after six months, you should contact your cleft palate clinic and ask for an appointment. At the clinic, the specialists will begin the process of learning why the expected improvement hasn't occurred. Their main task will be to find out if the initial surgery has provided your child with a palate that can close off the nose from the mouth.

The members of the clinic team will begin their evaluation by asking for your observations. For example, they will want to know about your child's eating and play activities? Does Aaron lose food into his nose when eating? Can Carol drink through a straw? Blow on a toy horn? Perhaps of more importance, they will want to know what sounds your child can make and what words he or she can say. They will be particularly interested in knowing if the child can make any consonant sounds that require closing off the nose from the mouth.

Team members will also listen to your daughter or son talk, noting if the child can blow air out of the mouth without losing air through the nose. They will also examine the mouth to see if the palate is intact and functioning. They may take X-ray movies of the mouth while the child speaks, blows, and swallows to see if the palate moves appropriately. Another procedure involves placing a tiny fiberoptic tube into the nose so that they can watch the palate move when the child talks.

Based on these observations and others, the team will make a decision about the cause of your child's speech problems. They may suggest additional surgery to improve the function of the palate or the use of speech prostheses to provide a better closure between the palate and the throat. (These procedures have been described in Chapter 3.) If it appears to the team that your child's palate is adequate for speech, then the solution to the problem is learning to use it appropriately. In this case, the team may suggest that you and your child work with a speech clinician.

When children are under three years of age, speech clinicians work with both the child and the parents. They usually begin the process by determining which sounds the child can and cannot make correctly. It is important to know this for several reasons. First, children with or without clefts do not learn to produce all consonants by age two or three. It may take several more years for them to master sounds such as *s*, *z, ch, sh, j, r,* and *l.* A three-year-old who doesn't make a reasonably good *m, n, p, b, d,* or *t,* however, may have a speech problem.

Second, by looking at the sounds a child produces correctly, it may be possible to determine the control he or she has over tongue movement or palatal closure. For example, the tongue tip elevates in the same way for "n" and "t." If three-year-old Adam makes the "n" in "no" correctly but makes a "k" instead of a "t" in the word "toe," his clinician knows that Adam didn't make the error because he can't elevate his tongue tip. Susan makes a correct "b" in the word "boy," which indicates that she can close off her nose from her mouth. Her difficulty in pronouncing the "t" in "toy" must be caused by a different problem.

The speech clinician needs a complete record of what a child can do so that the child's progress can be followed over time. As we have pointed out, all children, whether they have clefts or not, acquire articulation skills at different rates. That is, Chris may learn to make "t" and "b" by age two, "s" and "z" by age three, and "r" and "l" by age four, while Anna doesn't learn "s" and "z" until age four and "r" and "l" until age six. In both instances, the children are progressing at rates that are normal for them. The important thing is that both continue to progress. If a child's articulation patterns show no change over time, then there is reason for concern.

Finally, it is important for a professional observer to learn not only if a sound can be made correctly, but also whether it is *consistently* made correctly. If a child is not able to make the sound, our task is to help him or her learn to make it. Far more often, however, we find that children can make the sounds we are looking for, but only in some words or under particular circumstances. When this occurs, the task of the speech clinician is to help the child learn to use the correct sound in more words and under more circumstances.

How do speech clinicians help children learn to articulate correctly? In the following section, we will describe some of the most common methods used to achieve this goal.

Preschool Stage

Perhaps the most important way to help a child improve his or her speech is to make sure that speech is viewed as a useful and pleasurable activity. Once again, this means that parents and other adults should talk to the child and respond to speech efforts frequently, especially when both adults and child are having fun. Children with speech problems inevitably experience some frustration and failure in their efforts to be understood. It is extremely important that these negative experiences do not lead to discouragement and disinterest in speaking. If speech is important to a child and a source of pleasure, he or she will work hard at the task of learning to articulate correctly.

Another important function is helping the child to listen attentively to the correct speech of others. Activities that encourage this attention include looking at picture books and naming the things pictured (kitty, lamb, engine, ducks, dog) or making sounds associated with the pictures (meow, ba ba, etc.) and then having the child point to the correct picture. Parents might also provide names for things in the child's environment, for example, giving toys names that the child can recognize and use successfully (mimi = doll, baba = bear).

Sometimes we want children to watch as well as listen to the way we make sounds. On occasion, a child should be encouraged to watch an adult's face while a name is being said before repeating the name. Some speech clinicians suggest that there should be a mirror in the house hung at a low level so that a child can watch his or her own face while making sounds and words.

It is important that children learn about sounds and words by watching and listening to others, but it is also important that they listen to their own sounds and words. Whenever a child makes a good sound or a reasonably clear word, he or she should be made aware of it, be praised for the effort, and be given a chance to make the word again. When three-year-old Beth learned to say the word "cookie" correctly, her parents, Bill and Marilyn, found an appropriate picture in a magazine and taped it to the refrigerator door, where Beth could see it. Reminded of her success, Beth showed off her ability to say the new word, sometimes over and over again.

If all this sounds familiar, it's because most parents do these things naturally when trying to help their children learn to speak. The only difference is that they may need to do them more often and more consistently when their child is having difficulty learning to articulate.

At times, it may be necessary to do more than encourage a child or help him or her listen to speech. Parents may have to intervene in a more direct manner by trying to teach the child specific sounds. This, too, can be done in a variety of ways. Perhaps the simplest is to ask the child to imitate you: watch your mouth, listen carefully, and say the sound just the way you do. Parents do this all the time, and it often works, particularly for beginning sounds in words and for sounds that can be seen, that is, those that are made with the lips (such as *p, b, m*) or with the tongue tip (such as *t, d, n*). This approach works best if we know from previous observations that the child is able to bring the lips together or elevate the tongue.

A closely related approach is one in which we try to use a sound that the child makes correctly to help him or her with one made incorrectly. For example, Tommy could make the "m" sound in "mama" correctly but said "ah-ah" for "papa." His mother tried pairing the two words by having Tommy watch himself in the mirror while saying "mama" and then telling him to say "papa" so that it looks like "mama." It was not long before Tommy was able to say "papa" in a reasonably clear and correct way. As simple as such approaches appear, they can be very helpful in accomplishing our goals.

On occasion, it is necessary to teach a child to use lips and tongue in non-speech activities before trying to make sounds in words. For example, the speech clinician wanted Becky to learn to blow air out of her mouth and to start the blowing from different positions in her mouth. Becky's parents showed her how to make a cotton ball move on a table surface by putting her lips together, building up air pressure, and allowing it to burst out. Becky learned that she could do the same thing by putting her tongue in the *n* or *t* position or by starting the puff in the back of her mouth. Once Becky had learned these ways of producing puffs of air, her parents asked her to make words such as "pea," "tea," or "key" using these blowing positions.

Most speech clinicians find the task of teaching a child to make a new sound much less difficult than getting the child to use the new sound consistently. This learning progresses more slowly and takes longer to complete. The child must learn to make the correct sound in different words and in different positions within words; for example, Becky must be able to make the "t" sound in "tea" and in "cat." She must also be able to make the sound correctly in a word that is embedded in a sentence: "The cat drank the milk."

Finally, Becky must learn to make sounds correctly whenever she speaks. It is not enough to learn to make them only in specific words or in specific play activities. New sounds must become so much a part of Becky's life that she makes them when she is playing or eating, when she is inside the house or outside, when she is talking to her mother or to a playmate.

These are seemingly difficult tasks, but they can be learned. In this chapter, we have described only a few of the ways in which this learning is accomplished. Your speech clinician will provide valuable assistance to you and your child in pursuing the goal of using correct sounds consistently.

So far, our discussion of speech in the preschool years has focused on the development of articulation skills. This is appropriate since our goal is to have a child with a cleft palate producing intelligible speech by the time he or she starts school. The sounds produced may not be exactly like those of adults, but the child's speech will be understood.

In relation to the speech goals for children with clefts, it might be helpful to know what is expected from children without these problems during the preschool years. As a general guideline, we expect that by eighteen months of age, 25 percent of the words a child produces will be intelligible. By twenty-four months of age, 50 percent or more will be intelligible, and by thirty-six months, 75 to 100 percent of a child's words should be capable of being understood. If a child starts life with a condition such as cleft palate, which makes learning to articulate difficult, he or she may be up to a year behind in this schedule.

While children with cleft palate may be slower in learning articulation, we do not expect them to be behind in their language development. That is, we expect them to begin saying words at about one year of age and to be using words to obtain things by eighteen months. By age two, children should begin putting two or more words together ("daddy bye-bye," "more milk," "my dolly"), and by age three, they should be using short sentences that include subjects and verbs ("Baby eat cookie," "Mama fall down," "Doggy run"). By four years, a child with a cleft should be able to carry on a limited conversation and to use many forms of language (pronouns, past tense verbs, plural nouns, adjectives, etc.). Finally, we expect children with clefts to enter school with normal language skills and intelligible speech.

Bobby Stein went through the typical stages of speech development during his preschool years. Bobby was born with a cleft of the hard and soft palate. During his first few months of life, his parents, Sarah and Leonard, observed Bobby carefully to make sure that his speech was developing normally.

Bobby's palate was repaired when he was one year old, and six weeks later, Sarah Stein called the speech clinician at the cleft palate clinic to report that Bobby had begun to say words but that they sounded "funny." For example, he called his sister Susan "icky" and his toy dog "ee-ee." Sarah also noticed that Bobby said "mana" when she picked him up. The speech clinician commended her for her careful observations and encouraged Sarah and the rest of the family to respond to Bobby's words as if they were real.

During Bobby's second year, he began to use more words and to put words together in short sentences, although some of them still didn't sound quite right. (For example, he said "no my-my" for "go by-by.") His family was becoming concerned about his language development.

At this point, the speech clinician suggested that the Steins should try helping Bobby to improve his articulation. Sarah and Leonard, in consultation with the clinician, decided to work on the consonants *b* and *p*. As props to use in their work, they got Bobby a big rubber ball and gave his toy dog the name "Puppy."

Working with Bobby, the Steins quickly discovered that he could hear the difference between "Puppy" and "Mommy." They encouraged him to watch and listen carefully as they said "Puppy" and then to say the word himself. After a few days, Bobby could produce a word that sounded more like "Puppy" than "Mommy," although it still wasn't pronounced as an adult would pronounce it.

In the following weeks, Bobby learned to make other consonant sounds—*t, d, k, g*. They weren't perfect, but they did make his speech more intelligible. This was particularly helpful because his vocabulary was growing and he was using many more sentences now.

During the next year, Bobby's speech and language continued to develop. When he was four years old, his parents considered putting him in a preschool program. The speech clinician on the cleft palate team recommended that the Steins meet with the school's speech clinician before making a decision. The new clinician visited with Bobby and talked to the teachers in the preschool. They all agreed that Bobby would be able to handle the school program.

While Bobby was in preschool, his parents, his teacher, and the school speech clinician continued to work with him in an effort to achieve normal speech and language. At the end of the year, they met to review Bobby's progress and to discuss the advisability of his going to kindergarten in the fall. They agreed that Bobby's language skills were average or better, that he worked well with other children, and that his speech was 80 to 90 percent intelligible. There was no reason why he should not go to kindergarten.

Bobby got along well in kindergarten. Some of his classmates were aware that his speech sounded different, but Bobby's pleasant, friendly nature and the fact that the teacher treated him exactly as she did the other children seemed to convince them that the differences they heard were not important.

Later Stages of Speech Development

When your child enters school, a speech clinician employed by the school will be available to help with any speech problems. Actually, most school speech clinicians would like to know about your child well before he or she enters school. We strongly urge you to contact the speech clinician in the school your child will attend at least one year before that time. This specialist will want to talk to you about the development of your child's speech and language skills and become familiar with present and future plans for treatment. The speech clinician may ask your permission to contact your cleft palate team so that its members can share their records and plans.

After learning about your child's status and the progress that has been made, the school's speech clinician will meet with you and make suggestions about the best way to help your child. In most cases, you will be given one of the following reports: (1) Amy's speech development is well within normal limits, and we see no need for help from the speech clinician or other school personnel; (2) Eric's speech appears to be developing appropriately. We see no need for speech therapy at this time, but we would like to see the child once every three months to make sure that development continues; (3) We believe that Miriam would benefit from speech therapy at this time. Therapy goals will be to improve articulation of consonant sounds that she has trouble pronouncing, (for example) s, z, k, g. We would like to see Miriam three times a week for 20-minute sessions, and we request your participation in home activities that will assist the learning process. We will be contacting you regarding these activities in the coming weeks. The decision to have Miriam enrolled in speech therapy is up to you.

If the speech clinician believes that your child needs help and you decide that therapy is advisable, the therapy procedures will be explained to you. In most instances, work on the articulation of consonants will proceed in the same manner as that described for preschool children. Activities will be planned to help your child listen to speech sounds and to learn how to make correct sounds. In this stage, as in the earlier one, the big job will be to bring the child to the point where the correct sounds are made consistently and in all situations. The main difference between preschool and school therapy will be the level of accomplishment expected. The speech clinician will now want the child to make sounds that are more like those made by an adult. The specialist will not expect articulation exactly like an adult's while the child is in the first or second grade, but he or she will expect to see progress in that direction.

During the early school years, the condition of your child's teeth may be a factor in an attempt to achieve perfection in articulation. Children with clefts have many of the same dental problems that other children have. Their baby teeth erupt, fall out, and are replaced by permanent teeth during the same period of time that they are trying to perfect their speech. It is important to remember that all children learn to articulate under these conditions.

It is also true, however, that some children with clefts have unique dental problems, as we saw in Chapter 6. While these problems seldom prevent a child from learning to make consonants in the manner required for intelligible speech, they may make it more difficult to make the sounds exactly as adults do. Ultimately, the child's dental problems will be resolved to the point where they are not a handicap to the production of normal adult speech.

Nasal Sounds in Speech

Up to this point, we have assumed that children born with cleft palates have been treated surgically, that they can close off their noses from their mouths, and that their major speech problem is learning correct production of consonants. Another set of circumstances may occur. The surgical correction of the palate may produce a palate closure mechanism that allows the child to close off the nose from the mouth sufficiently so that he or she can learn to make consonants and produce intelligible speech, but the closure may not be complete. Some air may continue to leak out the nose, causing the child's speech to sound somewhat nasal.

Nasality in these circumstances may or may not be a matter for concern. The truth is that some nasality is present in the speech of many persons who do not have cleft palates and who are considered to have normal speech. If the nasal sound present in an individual with a cleft is within the range found in persons without clefts, it may not be a problem. If there is any question about its being considered a problem, however, an attempt should be made to decrease it.

There are three possible ways to deal with undesirable nasality. A surgeon may try to reconstruct the closure mechanism with the hope of decreasing the nasality, using the surgical procedures discussed in Chapter 3. Another option would be the insertion of a speech prosthesis, also described in Chapter 3. A prosthesis reduction program would then be used to reduce nasality and eventually eliminate the need for the prosthesis. A third approach involves working with a speech clinician to see if the child can learn to produce less nasal speech. This final approach is often tried before resorting to speech prostheses or surgery.

The decision to try reducing nasality by speech therapy is based on observations of speech and other diagnostic procedures. When these observations indicate that the child can decrease nasality under some set of circumstances, the speech clinician will try to help the child learn how to maintain this decrease in all speaking activities. The procedures used are very similar to those employed to help a child correct articulation errors: listening to sounds and recognizing the decrease in nasality; learning to produce words and sentences with this decreased level; perfecting the new skill until it is present in all speaking activities.

If speech therapy is not successful in reducing nasality, a speech prosthesis may be tried. As explained in an earlier chapter, these devices are designed to provide the child with a mechanism that allows complete closure between the nose and the mouth, thus eliminating the production of nasal speech.

Laura Gomez had problems with nasality that had not been reduced by therapy, so her doctors decided to try a speech bulb reduction program to improve her speech. Laura was fitted with a speech bulb that gave her complete closure between her mouth and nose. Then she worked with a speech therapist to produce non-nasal speech with the bulb in place. When she had mastered this, the prosthesis was slightly reduced in size. Now Laura's palate and throat walls had to move a little farther to produce good speech.

After several months of work, Laura succeeded in speaking normally with the smaller bulb. The size of the speech bulb was gradually reduced until Laura was finally able to produce non-nasal speech without the help of a prosthesis. The device had done its job in training Laura's palatal muscles to achieve closure and was now no longer needed.

In some cases, neither therapy nor the use of a speech prosthesis is successful, and surgery is the only option available. Through one of these three methods, nasality can almost always be eliminated or reduced to a level well within socially acceptable limits. The process may be tedious, but the results are impressive. With few exceptions, children born with clefts will enter adult life with acceptable speech.

Chapter 8
THE IMAGE IN THE MIRROR: HOW CLEFTS AFFECT SOCIAL AND PSYCHOLOGICAL DEVELOPMENT

All parents have high hopes and expectations for their children. They want them to develop a positive self-image, to be liked and make many friends, to do well in school, and to mature into well-adjusted, productive adults. Parents of children with clefts have these same hopes and dreams, but they often wonder whether their child's physical problems may limit the attainment of these goals. This question may have crossed your mind frequently since the birth of your "special" child.

As you have learned from the previous chapters of this book, all treatment of children with clefts has as its goal the achievement of acceptable facial structures and function in speech and hearing. Despite such treatment, however, some abnormalities in appearance and in speech will be carried into adulthood. Of course, as we well know, there are no perfect human beings. We all have our differences and imperfections, be they physical or behavioral. People with repaired clefts usually are no more or less flawed or different than the average adult in this less-than-perfect world.

How Parents React to a Cleft

No one can deny the initial shock and disappointment that

parents feel when their child is born with a cleft lip or palate. You were probably unprepared for the birth of a child with a defect and may have been unfamiliar with this particular defect, which is so noticeable in a newborn infant. Mixed with your early feelings of shock, pain, and guilt, there was probably concern about the effect that your reactions and the reactions of others might have on your child's psychological and social development.

Vicky Sloan responded in just this way when her daughter, Emma, was born with a bilateral cleft of the lip and palate. She had never seen a person with a cleft before and was deeply distressed when she saw her newborn daughter for the first time. After the inital shock was over, Vicky had all kinds of questions about Emma's future. How would people react to her daughter's appearance? Would she be teased by other children? Would she ever have any friends? What about Emma's ability to learn? Would the cleft have a drastic effect on her experiences in school?

Vicky's distress was normal and her concerns typical of most parents of children born with cleft. In many cases, parents go through a period of sadness and mourning after the birth of a child with a defect. These initial feelings are appropriate and expected, but professionals believe it is important that they do not last too long or become so extreme that they interfere with parents functioning as parents.

When you begin to understand the nature of your child's problem and the treatment that is available, the early anxiety, guilt, and other negative feelings should diminish. During this process, you should share your anxieties with the professionals treating your child so that they can help you learn about the defect and adjust to its existence. After the adjustment is made, you will be able to function comfortably as a parent, doing all the things that parents do for their children. In fact, research on families having children with clefts shows that parents are able to cope quite well and that the initial negative reactions do not have any long-term effect on parent-child relationships.

Growing Up With a Cleft

It seems clear that parents of children with clefts soon become comfortable with their roles and responsibilities as parents. But what about the children themselves? How do they cope with their physical defects? Let's begin by saying that we do not *expect* a child to have psychological or social problems because of a cleft lip or palate. This statement is based on the findings of a number of research studies that have investigated these areas. It would be realistic to say, however, that such children are at higher *risk* for psychosocial problems because of several factors.

If the cleft involves the lip, it is generally quite visible and may cause negative reactions in brothers and sisters, in schoolmates and teachers, and in others. If the palate is involved, there may be speech problems as well as frequent ear infections and perhaps hearing loss. These factors too could affect a child's psychological and social development. The long hospital stays early in a child's life and the resulting separation from parents could also create some behavioral and adjustment problems. As parents, you need to be aware of all these risk factors and to help your children deal with them.

In helping their children, parents also need to be aware of their own reactions, responses, and expectations. Parental beliefs influence children. A study done some years ago revealed that parents of children with cleft lip or palate see their children as less independent, aggressive, and confident than other young people.

Despite such beliefs, most professionals believe that there is no such thing as a "cleft palate personality." There are as many different personalities among children with clefts as there are among childern without this defect. By and large, young children and adolescents with clefts tend to have a self-image similar to those of other children.

It is not surprising, however, that people with clefts are sometimes less than totally satisfied with the appearance of their lips and teeth and with their speech performance. Some studies have suggested that adolescents with cleft lip and palate do report higher dissatisfaction with physical appearance than their peers without clefts. This seems to be especially true among young women, probably because of the importance of female physical attractiveness in our society.

One important factor in your child's social adjustment is coping with being teased. Teasing is one of the major concerns of parents, perhaps because it is something they cannot control. It is very likely that your child will at some time be teased by other children, just as Tony Andretti was when he started nursery school.

Although Tony was four, he had not had much contact with other children. He was an only child, and during his early years, he had spent a lot of time in the hospital or working with a therapist on speech problems. Now his speech was much improved, but he still had difficulty pronouncing some consonants. Although the cleft in his lip had been repaired for several years, the scar was still apparent and Tony's nostrils were unevenly shaped. During his first weeks at nursery school, some of the other children made comments on his appearance and asked persistent questions about what had happened to him. A few also began imitating his imperfect speech.

Tony felt bad about the teasing, but his parents had warned him that it might happen and prepared him to deal with it. He answered the questions about his appearance honestly and pretended that he didn't hear the kids who were imitating him. Even so, he came home in tears on more than one occasion and told his parents that he wasn't sure that he liked going to school.

Tony's parents had acted wisely in discussing teasing with their son before he started school. A child will be better able to respond to such an experience if parents explain that all children, with or without clefts, are teased at some time, just as they tease others. As adults, parents know that children can be brutal in their teasing and that they usually focus on some vulnerable point in others, usually something obvious such as appearance or speech. Such teasing hurts, but for children who have learned to feel good about themselves, it does not usually cause lasting damage. If a child like Tony grows up knowing that he is valued and loved, teasing about imperfections, which everyone has, will not destroy his self-image. Parents can help by making sure their child understands that a scarred lip or a speech flaw is only one small part of what makes a whole person.

We believe that children with clefts should be given a simple explanation of their defect as soon as they are old enough to ask questions or to be questioned by playmates. Some parents hesitate to tell their children because they fear it may make them "feel different." But even very young children already know that something about them is different because of the many doctors involved in their care. When Steven was four, a playmate told him he "talked funny" and "looked funny." Steven's response was, "I know—that's why I go to see all those doctors. They're helping me to get better."

Another concern of parents is academic achievement. In general, you can expect achievement to be within normal limits. There have been no studies indicating that persons with clefts have less intelligence than persons without clefts. Certain studies, however, have suggested that some children with cleft palate achieve at lower levels and may have specific learning disabilities. Experts think that such difficulties are often related to speech and hearing problems. If these problems are being corrected, then the learning handicaps should also disappear.

Becoming Adults

When children with clefts become adults, some continue to be concerned about their appearance and speech. A study that interviewed adults with cleft lip and palate showed that while such concerns still existed, the respondents generally felt that their clefts had had little effect in their adult lives. The people in this study reported a high degree of satisfaction with their jobs and their marriages. In a larger study using questionnaires with adults having cleft lip and palate, only minor differences were found between those questioned and people without clefts in areas such as marriage, education, vocation, and general social factors. No studies suggest that there is a high rate of emotional problems among people with clefts.

Although people with clefts generally make a good social and psychological adjustment, this does not mean that some individuals may not have significant problems. If such problems exist, it is important to identify them and to obtain professional help, just as is done in other areas of concern related to clefts. Fortunately, there are many available resources if assistance is needed. Your interdisciplinary team will probably include a psychologist or social worker who can identify potential problems and recommend appropriate professional help.

Chapter 9

CAN THIS HAP-PEN AGAIN? THE IMPORTANCE OF GENETIC COUNSELING

A great deal of research is currently being done on the causes of cleft lip and palate. Researchers are attempting to get a better understanding of the genetic component of the defect and the developmental mechanisms that produce clefting. In studying this birth defect and many others, scientists are making use of knowledge about human genetics that has been gained in recent years. In the future it may be possible to pinpoint the exact cause of clefting and even to make changes in genetic material that would prevent this defect from occurring in some cases. Although we don't have such knowledge today, we do have a better understanding of why clefts occur in families and whether they will be likely to occur again. This information is available to you through genetic counseling.

Will It Happen Again?

A genetic counselor can help you answer a question that has probably been on your mind since your child was born: If I have other children, will they have clefts too? In a real sense, parents learn about their own genetic makeup only through their children. They usually do not know that they have a genetic tendency for a certain disorder until they produce a child with that disorder. When this happens, it is too late to make a decision about that particular child, but genetic counseling can help you make decisions about future children. By examining your child and analyzing your family history, a counselor can give you information on the probable causes of the cleft and on the likelihood of its occurring again.

One cause of clefts can be traced to problems with a single gene inherited by a child. There are a number of hereditary or congenital disorders in which several defects, including clefting, tend to appear together. The medical term for such a group of symptoms is "syndrome," which means "running together." Since some of these syndromes are caused by defects in a single gene, we know something about the way they are transmitted and the genetic risk of their reappearing in a family. When the Allens went in for genetic counseling, they found out that the risk in their family was relatively high.

Richard Allen was two years old when he and his parents, Barbara and Ned, were first seen in the cleft palate clinic. Richard, who had been born with cleft lip and palate, was the only child of two supposedly normal parents. Barbara and Ned wanted to have more children, but they were concerned about the possibility of clefting occurring again in their family.

When the Allens were evaluated by the genetic counselor, Ned was found to have small depressions or pits on the inside of his lower lip. His son had the same small pits. This information revealed a great deal about the cause of Richard's cleft and the probability of other children in the family having the problem. The presence of the lip pits in both parent and child indicated a genetic syndrome that is strongly associated with clefting. Because of this, Richard's cleft had a much larger hereditary component than isolated cleft lip and palate. His chance of being born with the defect had been about 50 percent, and any other children the Allens might have would have the same risk.

In the Allen family, a single defective gene was probably the cause of the syndrome that produced Richard's cleft. In a very small number of cases, clefting may also be associated with an abnormal chromosome condition, such as an extra chromosome or a partially missing one. People with this kind of problem are usually born with a number of obvious defects, of which clefting is among the least serious.

Clefts that are the result of syndromes or abnormal chromosomes account for a small percentage of all persons born with cleft lip and palate. In the large majority of cases, the defect is caused not by genetic problems alone but by a combination of genetic and environmental factors. Researchers have learned that these "multifactorial" cases can be separated into two different categories. One category is made up of clefts that occur in families. *Familial clefts* affect parents, brothers and sisters, or other close relatives. The other category of multifactorial clefts is referred to as *sporadic*. It includes isolated cases of cleft lip and palate in which no other close relatives have the defect. Studies have shown that more than 80 percent of all clefts fall into the sporadic category.

By analyzing your family history, a genetic counselor can usually tell you whether your child's cleft is of the familial or sporadic type. Based on this information, the counselor can also give you some statistics on the probability of having other children born with clefts. Here are some of the possibilities: If both parents are normal and have one child with a cleft, the chances for the next child to be born with a cleft are less than 3 percent (that is, less than 3 chances out of 100). If one parent has a cleft, the chance for the first child to have a cleft is still under 3 percent. If the first child in this family is born with a cleft, however, the chance for the next child to have the defect rises to approximately 15 percent. Two normal parents whose first two children have clefts also have a 15 percent chance of bearing a third child with the defect. As you can see, the chances are higher in these cases of familial clefts than they are when only one family member has the defect.

Although these risk figures apply to the majority of families with clefts, they may not apply to you. It cannot be overemphasized that each case is unique. Many causal factors are involved, and they can affect each person somewhat differently. That's why it is important that you and your family seek genetic counseling to learn about your specific situation.

Genetic counseling can also help to relieve the guilt felt by many parents of children with clefts. These parents often believe that they are entirely responsible for their child's problem; something they did must have caused the clefting. Such beliefs create a burden of guilt that can be overwhelming. This is another reason why getting the correct information on the cause of clefting in a family is so important. When parents learn that their child's cleft was probably caused by a combination of factors and that none of these factors was under their control, guilty feelings are eased and they are able to make decisions about the future.

Melissa Quinley had harbored secret feelings of guilt ever since her two-year-old son, Ryan, was born with a cleft lip. She remembered being told that her great grandfather's brother had had a cleft of some kind, and she felt that her family's genes were responsible for Ryan's cleft. Now Melissa was pregnant again, and she was afraid that the child she was carrying would also be born with a cleft.

In her fourth month of pregnancy, Melissa and her husband, Jim, came to the cleft palate clinic requesting some kind of test that would tell whether their unborn child had the defect. They were told that an ultrasound examination might be able to reveal a cleft lip but that genetic counseling would be more helpful in answering their questions.

After meeting with the genetic counselor, Melissa was relieved to learn she was not the cause of Ryan's cleft. The one instance of clefting in her family was too far in the past to have any significance. Melissa's chances of having a normal baby were greater than 97 percent, just the same as those of any parent who has had one child with a cleft. Ryan is now ten years old and doing just fine. He has two younger brothers and a sister born without clefts.

Mike Stone's case also shows how genetic counseling can clear up confusion and help in making plans for the future. Mike was the second child of parents who had died in an automobile accident when he was five. Both of his parents had clefts, and Mike was born with a cleft lip and palate. His older brother did not have the defect. Mike's clefts had been repaired, and his speech was excellent. Because of an unstable family situation, however, Mike had not been seen regularly by a cleft palate team during his childhood. Now, at age 25, he had come in for interdisciplinary evaluation and genetic counseling.

Mike told the counselor that he assumed his chance of having children with clefts was 75 percent since he and both his parents had the defect—three out of the four members of his family. This assumption had had a significant effect on his life so far. Mike reported a definite reluctance to establish relationships and to consider marriage since he believed that his risk of having children with clefts was so high. Based on his family history, however, his risk did not exceed 15 percent, assuming that he married a woman who did not have a cleft. This figure was much lower than the one that Mike had accepted for so many years. After talking to a genetic counselor, Mike felt that he now understood his situation and was better prepared to make decisions in the future.

Mike's story and the others told here illustrate the importance of thorough family evaluation by a genetic counselor to provide the most accurate information. That information will enable family members to better understand what has caused the clefting and what might happen in the future.

. . . .
. . . .
. . . .
. . . .
. . . .
. . . .

Chapter 10
A FINAL
WORD—
OPTIMISM

For all the readers of this book—parents and others interested in knowing more about cleft lip and palate—we hope that one word has come through loudly and clearly. That word is *optimism.*

In the last several years, surgeons, dentists, speech clinicians, and other professionals have learned much and have made great advances in treating cleft lip and palate. Research now underway will continue to increase our understanding of the disorder and improve our care of people with clefts. Even with the treatment currently available, however, it is safe to say that we can expect a child with cleft lip and palate to develop into adulthood with very acceptable appearance, dental function, and communication and social skills. Of course, people with repaired clefts will not be perfect in every respect. There are imperfections in all of us. Their chances for educational, vocational, and social achievement, however, should be just as great as those of people without clefts.

The Cost of Care

Optimism, therefore, is justified, but it does not come without cost. Some of the cost must be paid in very real dollars and cents. In any disorder involving multiple procedures carried out over a long period of time, treatment can be expensive. Cleft lip and palate is no exception. Both parents and medical personnel want to keep costs down while providing the most beneficial treatment for the child. There are ways in which this can be done.

First, the prevention of dental problems with regular professional care and excellent oral hygiene cannot be overemphasized. A clean mouth with few, if any, cavities is an important foundation for successful dental and surgical procedures. Preventive dental care is an inexpensive way to avoid some very expensive problems in the future.

Second, periodic evaluation by an interdisciplinary team is important in planning the most appropriate treatment for your child over time. The team approach is not only the most beneficial but also the most efficient and cost-effective way to achieve the best possible results.

Third, the heavy financial burden of paying for the care of cleft lip and palate treatment can be eased by assistance from various outside sources. Third-party payers such as medical and dental insurance plans are the primary sources for helping with diagnostic and treatment services. Although most plans cover individual treatments such as palate surgery, some do not pay for interdisciplinary procedures involving dental, hearing, and speech problems. An effort is being made on a national level to impress upon medical/dental insurers that the cost of such procedures is directly related to the original cleft and that it should be covered.

In addition to insurance plans, there are public support programs that can help with treatment costs. Every state has a federally funded program that provides funds for treating a variety of disorders in children, including cleft lip and palate. Costs typically are shared between the program and the family. For specific information regarding these programs, contact the Department of Health or Human Services in your state. There are also a number of other support programs for which individual families may qualify. These include state and county medical assistance, vocational rehabilitation, and treatment at public and private teaching institutions, to name only a few.

With help from these different sources, the cost of treatment can usually be handled by most families. While we would certainly like to see more support funds available for people with cleft lip and palate, cost alone should not prevent you from receiving the best possible care for your child.

Commitment to the Best Care

The best possible care will also require commitment—commitment on the part of the child, of parents and other family members, and of the interdisciplinary team. Such commitment is vital considering the long-range nature of treatment for cleft lip and palate. During the many years of surgical and dental repairs, speech therapy, and other procedures, all involved must continue to work toward the ultimate goals of the treatment.

We firmly believe that the interdisciplinary approach is the key to lasting commitment and optimal care. We encourage parents to become acquainted with their interdisciplinary teams as soon as possible in the course of treatment. In this way, you will be able to address early questions about your child's condition and future problems to the appropriate team member.

At this period and throughout treatment, a harmonious relationship and effective communication between your family and the interdisciplinary clinic team are essential. With this kind of cooperation and commitment, you can be sure that your child will receive the very best care and will have every chance to live a normal, productive life.

GLOSSARY

Alveolar process. The part of the bony upper jaw that contains teeth; also called the alveolar ridge.

Arch collapse. The displacement of sections of the alveolar process caused by the existence of clefts.

Articulation. The process of forming speech sounds.

Audiologist. A professional who specializes in the identification and treatment of hearing problems.

Bilateral cleft. A cleft that occurs on both sides of the lip.

Chromosomes. Tiny threads of the genetic material DNA, contained within human cells. Each chromosome is made up of many different genes.

Cleft. A split or opening in the lip or palate.

Complete cleft. A cleft that extends through the whole of the affected mouth structure.

Crossbite. A condition in which some of the upper teeth are positioned inside the lower teeth (in the direction of the tongue). Crossbite results from the displacement of individual teeth in the bony upper jaw segments.

Deciduous teeth. Primary or baby teeth.

Eustachian tube. The tube that connects the middle ear to the back of the throat.

Familial clefts. Clefts that affect several close relatives in the same family.

Fistula. An abnormal opening.

Gene. One of the sections of DNA that make up a chromosome. A gene is the basic unit of heredity. Genes inherited from parents determine a child's physical characteristics.

Genetic counselor. A specialist who can advise parents about the risk of having children with clefts or other birth defects.

Hard palate. The hard, bony part of the roof of the mouth.

Interdisciplinary approach. A method of treating cleft lip and palate in which several medical, dental, speech, and hearing specialists work together, coordinating their efforts and planning treatment.

Larynx. A structure located at the top of the trachea that produces sound; also called the voice box.

Lateral maxillary segments. The two side segments of the bony upper jaw.

Levator muscles. Muscles that lift or elevate, such as the levator muscles of the soft palate.

Mandible. The movable lower jaw.

Maxilla. The bony upper jaw.

Mixed dentition phase. The period during which a child has some deciduous teeth and some permanent teeth.

Myringotomy. A procedure in which a small needle is inserted through the eardrum to drain off excess fluid.

Nasality. A nasal sound in speech, often found in people with cleft palates.

Occlusion. The relationship between the upper and lower teeth when they are in contact; also known as bite.

Orthodontist. A dental specialist who uses braces and other appliances to reposition teeth or jaw segments.

Otitis media. An inflammation of the middle ear caused by infections, allergies, or improper functioning of the eustachian tube.

Otolaryngologist. A medical specialist who is concerned with diseases and conditions of the ear, nose, and throat.

Overbite. The normal relationship in which the teeth in the upper jaw slightly overlap those in the lower jaw.

Overjet. The normal relationship in which the teeth in the upper jaw are slightly in front of those in the lower jaw.

Palatal lengthening. A surgical procedure in which tissue from the front part of the mouth is moved back to lengthen it; also known as palatal pushback.

Palatal lift. A device inserted into the mouth that raises the soft palate so that it contacts the back wall of the throat, improving closure; often used as a training device in speech therapy.

Palate. The roof of the mouth, made up of the hard and soft palates.

Partial cleft. A cleft that extends through part of the affected mouth structure.

Pediatric dentist. A dentist specializing in the dental care of children.

Pharyngeal. Relating to the pharynx or back of the throat.

Pharyngeal flap surgery. A procedure in which the surgeon creates a flap or bridge of tissue that connects the soft palate to the back wall of the throat to improve closure.

Pharyngeal augmentation. Pieces of tissue or artificial substances placed in the back wall of the throat to reduce the distance that the soft palate must move to achieve closure.

Premaxilla. The front central section of the bony upper jaw, somewhat triangular in shape. The premaxilla contains the four upper front teeth.

Pressure consonants. Those consonants that require a buildup of pressure in the mouth. People with cleft palate often find these consonants difficult to produce.

Primary surgery. The initial surgery to repair a cleft lip or palate.

Prosthodontist. A dental specialist who replaces missing teeth with partial dentures or fixed bridges.

Resonators. Cavities such as the mouth, nose, and throat that can be used to change the nature of sound produced by the larynx. By changing the openings of these cavities and their size and shape, we make different vowels.

Secondary surgery. Surgery done after primary surgery to improve appearance or to correct additional problems.

Speech bulb. A device that occupies space in the back of the throat so that the throat walls have to move only a short distance to close off the mouth from the nose; often used as a training device to improve speech.

Speech clinician. A professional whose speciality is the identification and treatment of speech problems; also known as a speech-language pathologist.

Speech prothesis. A device inserted into the mouth to achieve closure; often used as a training device to improve speech.

Sporadic clefts. Isolated cases of cleft lip and palate affecting only one member of a family.

Trachea. A tube that carries air to and from the lungs. The larynx is located at the top of the trachea..

Unilateral cleft. A cleft that occurs on only one side of the lip.

Uvula. The small piece of tissue connected to the soft palate that hangs down in the back of the throat.

Velopharyngeal closure. The separation between the mouth and nose made when the soft palate is raised to contact the back wall of the throat. Closure is necessary for speech, blowing, and swallowing.

Ventilation tube. A small tube inserted into the eardrum to allow air to reach the middle ear.

Vocal folds. Two lip-like structures inside the larynx that vibrate when air from the lungs is forced through them, producing sound.

HELPFUL ORGANIZATIONS

National Organizations

American Cleft Palate Association

The American Cleft Palate Association (ACPA) was established in 1943 for the purpose of stimulating "specialist and public interest in, and a more exact knowledge and improved practice of, the science and art of the rehabilitation of persons with cleft palate and associated anomalies" (Preamble of the ACPA Constitution, 1987). The organization's membership is made up of people from a variety of professional backgrounds: medicine, speech and hearing, dental specialties, psychology, social work, nutrition, nursing, and others. All are interested in improving the welfare of persons with cleft palate.

ACPA National Office
1218 Grandview Avenue
University of Pittsburgh
Pittsburgh, PA 15211
(412) 481-1376

Cleft Palate Foundation

Established in 1973, the Cleft Palate Foundation (CPF) has as its primary purpose informing and educating public and professional people about cleft palate and other craniofacial deformities. The foundation's main activities include sponsoring informational programs intended to encourage, assist, and contribute to research in the field. These activities are conducted in cooperation with the American Cleft Palate Association.

Cleft Palate Foundation, Inc.
1218 Grandview Avenue
University of Pittsburgh
Pittsburgh, PA 15211
(412) 481-1376

National Cleft Palate Association

Established in 1984, the National Cleft Palate Association (NCPA) is an organization of parents, families, and individuals with clefts. Its stated goal is the advancement of the health, welfare, and education of children and adults with cleft lip and palate and related craniofacial anomalies. NCPA activities include

— educating the public about cleft lip and palate and the resources available to affected individuals
— assisting in the development of local parent-patient support groups
— serving as an advocate for affected individuals and their families, including providing assistance with legislative review of insurance coverage
— promoting research about cleft lip and palate
— promoting cooperative efforts with the American Cleft Palate Association, the Cleft Palate Foundation, and other professional organizations.

National Cleft Palate Association
1218 Grandview Avenue
University of Pittsburgh
Pittsburgh, PA 15211
1-800-24-CLEFT

There is a close affiliation and cooperation between the three national organizations listed here. Although each has its special focus and purpose, all three exist to contribute to the welfare of persons with cleft lip and palate.

Help 24 Hours a Day

Cleft Line 1-800-24-CLEFT

This 24-hour telephone service provides information and referrals for the public or professionals. The Cleft Line was developed by the Cleft Palate Foundation in cooperation with the National Cleft Palate Association. (In Pennsylvania, call 1-800-23-CLEFT.)

State and Local Resources

Many states, counties, and cities have active parent-patient support groups. Some are affiliated with interdisciplinary teams at hospitals or clinics; most, however, function independently from specific teams. The National Cleft Palate Association can help by providing information about existing groups in your area or guidance in establishing new groups. Call Cleft Line for this information.

Information about interdisciplinary teams in your area and financial assistance should be available by contacting one or more of the following:

—your state's Department of Health or Department of Human Services. These agencies administer the funds provided by a national program called Maternal and Child Health Services. State programs that are part of this plan were formerly known as Crippled Children's Services but are now listed under a variety of other names. Vocational Rehabilitation Programs in your area may also be a source of help.

—Your county's Health and Human Services Department. This agency can be a resource for nutritional, dental, and public-health nursing services.

—Special national, state, and local financial assistance programs for which you may qualify. These might include Medical Assistance Programs, Indian Health Services, and programs sponsored by local university or teaching hospitals. All may cover, or substantially reduce, the costs of evaluation and treatment.

The interdisciplinary clinic that you attend may also have resources to help you in paying for evaluation and treatment. Other sources of help are private and public insurance plans, which are increasingly contributing to evaluation and treatment costs incurred by families. Several states have passed legislation that requires medical/dental insurance plans to assume a larger role in paying for the comprehensive treatment of persons with cleft lip and palate.

SUGGESTED READING

Books about Speech and Language

Brookshire, B., Lynch, J., and Fox, D. *A Parent-Child Palate Curriculum. Developing Speech and Language.* CC Publications, Tigard, Oregon, 1980.
Presents a speech and language curriculum for children from birth through 36 months. It suggests specific goals and activities designed to help children reach these goals. The book contains many practical suggestions and is very readable.

deVillers, Peter and Jill. *Early Language.* Harvard University Press, Cambridge, Massachusetts, 1979.
Describes the development of speech and language in children. The book does not deal specifically with children who have clefts, but the information it contains is applicable to them. Although it is used as a textbook in university courses, it is not technical and is easy to read.

McWilliams, B., Morris, H., and Shelton, R. *Cleft Palate Speech.* C. V. Mosby Company, St. Louis, Missouri, 1984.
This textbook is used in university courses on the speech and hearing problems associated with cleft palate. It is somewhat technical, but readable. It contains chapters on speech and hearing, as well as on surgical and dental problems associated with clefts.

Information on Feeding and Nutritional Needs

Bennett, V. *Feeding Young Children with Cleft Lip and Palate*. A pamphlet published by the Minnesota Dietetic Association, 1821 University Avenue, Suite S-280, St. Paul, MN 55104.
A very practical guide to feeding children with clefts.

Farnan, S. "Nutrition and Feeding of Children with Cleft Palate." *Nutrition News* March/April 1988:1–4.
An excellent article on nutrition needs published in a magazine that should be available in many public libraries.

Feeding Your Special Baby. A pamphlet published by the Center for Craniofacial Anomalies, University of Illinois at Chicago, 809 S. Wood Street, Chicago, ILL 60680.
Another practical guide, focusing on feeding during the first six months.

Advice on Special Concerns and Problems

Brown, H. "Different? I'm Not Different." *Cleft Palate Journal* 20 (1983):85–86.

Clifford, E. *The Cleft Palate Experience*. C. C. Thomas Publishers, Springfield, Illinois, 1987.

Clifford, C. "Why Are They So Normal?" *Cleft Palate Journal* 20 (1983):83–84.

MacDonald, Susan Kelley, "Parental Needs and Professional Responses: A Parental Perspective." *Cleft Palate Journal* 16 (1979):188–192.

"Teasing and the Disabled Child." *The Exceptional Parent* April 1985:36–44.

The magazines and books listed here should be available in university libraries and some public libraries. *The Cleft Palate Journal* contains numerous articles related to clefts, though many are quite technical.

INDEX

INDEX

Academic achievement. *See* Psychosocial issues

Adenoids, diagram, 76

Adjustment. *See* Psychosocial issues

Alveolar process (ridge): defined, 55, 115; growth of, 55; in clefts, 61–64; treatment in clefts, 66–67

American Cleft Palate Association, 119

Arch collapse: defined, 115; diagrams: bilateral, 62; unilateral, 63; in clefts, described, 61–64, *See also* Crossbite

Articulation (speech): early development, 83; parents' role in development of, 94–95; treatment: preschool, 94–95; later, 95–96. *See also* Speech-language development

Audiologist: defined, 115; described, 14, 52

Bone graft: examples of, 68, 73; for clefts, 67; reasons for, 67

Bottle feeding, types of, 40

Breastfeeding, possibility of, 40

Chromosomes: abnormality as cause of clefting, 106–7; defined, 11, 115

Cleft Line, 121

Cleft Palate Foundation, 119–20

Clefting: chromosomal, 11, 107; development of, 5–10; frequency of, 10; genetic, 11; genetic and environmental, 12, 107; in syndromes, 106

Closure (speech). *See* Velopharyngeal closure

Consonants: diagrams, 80; in speech, described, 79. *See also* Speech/language development

Cost: insurance, 112; of care, 111–12; of public programs, 112–13

Crossbite (dental): bilateral, 61–62; unilateral, 61–63; described, 61; defined, 115. *See also* Arch collapse

Deciduous (baby) teeth. *See* Teeth

Dental health, importance of, 65

Dental treatment: early preventive care, 64–65; importance of, 64; pediatric dentistry, 64; team, 72–74

Ear: drum, 46–47; function, 46–47;
    identification of problems,
    50–52; normal structure of,
    45–46; parts of outer, 45;
    middle, 46; inner, 46; problems
    in clefting, 47–48; treatment of,
    48–50
Earaches, 45
Early speech concerns, possible
    treatment, 88–89, 93
Embryology (womb development),
    lip and palate, nose, 5–8
Emotional problems, in persons
    with clefts, 104
Eustachian tube (auditory tube):
    defined, 115; described, 45–46;
    function, 46

Familial clefts, 107
Family history, use of in genetic
    counseling, 107
Feeding: after surgery, 43; bottles
    and nipples used in, 40;
    concerns, 14, 39–40, 43;
    position, 40–41; solids, 42
Fistulae: defined, 116; described,
    34–35

Genes: defined, 11, 116; multiple
    gene cause of clefting, 107;
    single gene cause of clefting,
    106
Genetic counseling, 105–9; and
    cause of clefts, 106–7; effect of,
    108–9; family history in, 106–7;
    importance of, 105
Genetic counselor: defined, 116;
    role of, 105–6
Genetic risks, for clefting, 107
Guilt, feelings of, 100, 108
Gum ridge. See Alveolar process

Hard palate: cleft, 6–11;
    development of, 6–7; normal, 8.
    See also Surgery, palate

Hearing: early concerns, 14–15;
    loss of, 50–54; parents'
    identification of problems with,
    50–53; structures used for,
    45–47

Incisive foramen, defined, 8
Interdisciplinary care: dental team,
    72–74; importance of, 16–17,
    113

Jaws: growth and development of,
    55; structure of, 55. See also
    Mandible, Maxilla

Language: defined, 82; effect of
    clefts on, 84–85; learning of,
    82–83, 93; parents' contribution
    in learning of, 83–84. See also
    Speech/language
Larynx: defined, 116; described,
    76; diagram, 76
Lip: asymmetry of, 27; cleft, 6, 8,
    10, 18; development of, 5–6;
    growth of, 27; normal, 7; pits,
    106; normal, 7. See also Surgery,
    lip
Loudness (speech), in cleft palate
    speakers, 77
Lungs, function of in speech, 77

Mandible: defined, 116; described,
    56; function of, 56; growth of,
    60
Maxilla (upper jaw): defined, 116;
    diagnosis, 56; growth of, 60;
    parts of, 55
Mixed dentition, timing, 58–59
Multifactorial inheritance, 107
Myringotomy: defined, 116;
    described, 49

Nasal structures. See Nose
Nasality: in speech, 79; treatment
    for, 97–98

National Cleft Palate Association, 120

Nose: development of, 5–6; nostril shape, 23; sugery, 22

Nutrition, importance of, 39

Obturator, 35

Occlusion (dental bite): defined, 116; described, 56–57, 59; effects of clefts on, 61–64; in permanent teeth, 59; in primary teeth, 57

Oral surgeon: role of, 15. *See also* Oral surgery

Oral surgery: concerns of, 67; interaction with orthodontist, 67–69; jaw surgery timing, 69–71; timing of treatment, 67

Organizations, for families with cleft palate: national, 119–21; state and local, 121–22

Orthodontics: concerns of, 65–66; interaction with oral surgeon, 67–69; timing of treatment, 66

Orthodontist: defined, 116; role of, 15. *See also* Orthodontics

Ossicles (ear bones), described, 45

Otitis media: chronic, 47–48; defined, 47, 116; treatment for, 48–50. *See also* Ear

Otolaryngologist: defined, 19, 117; role of, 14

Overbite, defined, 56–57

Overjet, defined, 56–57

Palatal lengthening, described, 34

Palatal lift: closure with, 35–36; defined, 35–36

Palate: clefts, 6–7, 9–10; development of, 6–7; normal, 8. *See also* Surgery, palate

Palate surgery. *See* Surgery, palate

Parents: expectations of psychological development, 99, 101; involvement and commitment of, 113; reactions to birth of children with cleft palate, 99–100

Pediatric dentist: preventive treatment and, 64–65; role of, 15

Pediatric surgeon, defined, 19

Pharyngeal augmentation, described, 34

Pharyngeal flap: defined, 33; described, 33; diagram of, 33

Pitch (speech), in cleft palate speakers, 77

Plastic and reconstructive surgeon, defined, 19

Premaxilla: in bilateral clefts, 61; defined, 117; described, 55; diagrams, 56, 57, 58, 62; teeth in, 59

Primary palate: clefts involving, 8–10; defined, 5; diagrams, 6, 8; formation of, 5–6

Prostheses (speech): closure with, 35–36; diagram of, 36; reasons for, 35; types of, 35

Prosthodontist: concerns of, 71; defined, 117; interaction with orthodontist, 72–75; role of, 15; treatment by, 71–72

Psychologist, on teams, 104

Psychosocial issues: academic achievement, 103; adjustment, 102; identification and treatment of, 104; parental responses, 103; and risk for problems, 101; self-image, 101

Quality (speech), in cleft palate speakers, 77

Research: in clefting, 111; in psychosocial aspects, 100–101, 103–4

Resources: for help, 119–22, *See also* Organizations

Resonators: defined, 118; described, 77–78; diagram, 78; importance in speech, 79

Self-image. *See* Psychosocial issues
Secondary palate: clefts of, 9–11; defined, 5, 9; diagrams of, 6, 8; formation of, 5–10
Social worker, on teams, 104
Soft palate: development of, 6–10; function of, 30–31, 76, 79–81; muscles in, 30; normal, 7, 8
Solids, in feeding, 42
Speech: and consonant production, 79–81; defined, 75; effects of clefting on, 84–86, 86–87; structures used to produce, 76–77; after surgery, 87–88, 90–96; and vowel production, 77–79
Speech bulb: closure with, 35–36; defined, 35; and reduction programs, 98
Speech-language clinician (pathologist, therapist); and articulation treatment, 90–96; function of, 85–86, 88–89; role of, 16
Speech/language development, 15–16, 82–87. *See also* Speech, Speech/language problems
Speech/language problems: described, 15–16, 86; after surgery, 87; treatment for, 88–98. *See also* Speech, Speech/language development, Speech treatment
Speech treatment: early, 88–89; preschool, 90; speech bulb, 98; surgery, 98; therapy, 97–98
Sporadic clefts, 107
Submucous cleft, defined, 10
Sucking, problems, 39–40
Surgery, lip: diagrams, 21, 24; examples of, 20–28; photos (before and after), 22–23, 25–26;

revisions, 24–28; timing, 13–14, 20
Surgery, palate: diagrams, 31; goals of, 29; revisions, 32; secondary, 32–35; timing, 14, 29; types, 29–31
Swallowing, 40
Syndrome: defined, 106; importance of identifying, 106–7

Team care. *See* Interdisciplinary care
Teasing, coping with, 102–3
Teeth: development of, 55–60; effects of clefts on, 15, 60–64; names of deciduous (primary), 56–57; names of permanent (secondary), 58
Tonsils, diagram, 76
Trachea: defined, 118; diagram, 76
Treatment: advancement in techniques, 111; cost, 111–12; dental, 64; goal of, 111; oral surgery, 66–69; orthodontic, 65–66, 68–70; prosthodontic, 35–37, 71–72; speech, 88–98; surgery, 19–35

Uvula: defined, 118; development of, 9

Velopharyngeal closure: defined, 118; importance in speech, 78–81; treatment to improve, 30–35, 35–37, 88–98
Ventilation tubes: defined, 49, 118
Vocal folds: defined, 118; described, 76; function of, 76–77
Vowels: diagram, 78; in speech described, 77. *See also* Speech/language development

Weaning, timing, 42

KARLIND MOLLER is professor and director of the Cleft Palate Maxillofacial and Craniofacial Clinics in the School of Dentistry at the University of Minnesota. Active in the community as well as in the University, Moller has served on several committees for the Minnesota Speech and Hearing Association and the American Cleft Palate Association. In 1985, he received the Outstanding Clinical Achievement Award from the Minnesota Speech, Language, and Hearing Association and the American Speech and Hearing Foundation. Moller earned his M.A. and Ph.D. at the University of Minnesota. His editorial consultantships include the *Journal of Speech and Hearing Disorders* and the *Cleft Palate Journal*, and he has published in the *Journal of Speech and Hearing Research*, the *Journal of Prosthetic Dentistry*, and the *Journal of Craniofacial Genetics and Developmental Biology*.

CLARK STARR is a professor at the University of Minnesota and a consultant to the University Cleft Palate Maxillofacial Clinic. He teaches, conducts research, and supervises clinical programs in the Department of Communication Disorders, where he has served as chairman and director of graduate studies. He has published in the *Cleft Palate Journal*, the *Journal of Speech and Hearing Research*, the *Journal of Speech and Hearing Disorders*, *Human Communication*, and *Folia Phoniatrica*, and has contributed chapters to books on cleft palate. He is a Fellow in the American Speech, Language and Hearing Association and a member of the American Cleft Palate Association and the International Association of Logopedics. He received a Ph.D. in speech pathology from Northwestern University in 1956.

SYLVIA A. JOHNSON is an editor and writer of books for young people; she is employed at Lerner Publications in Minneapolis, and works as a freelancer as well. An M.A. in English from the University of Illinois, Johnson has collaborated with writers in the fields of anthropology, archaeology, botany, behavioral biology, entomology, psychiatry, and many other disciplines. She has written and edited books which received awards from the National Science Teachers Association, the New York Academy of Sciences, and the Children's Book Council.